CW00722002

THE
SLIMMER'S YEAR

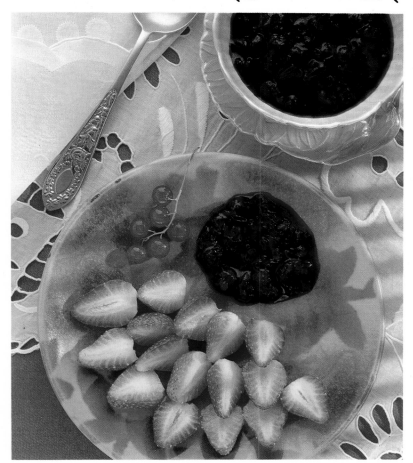

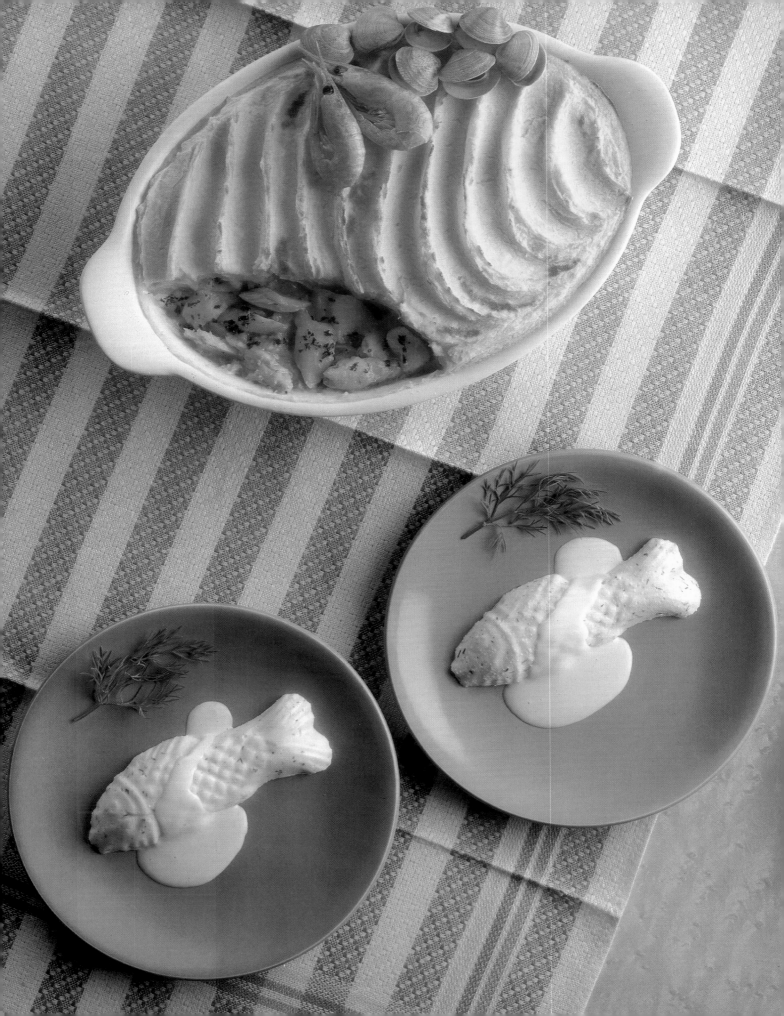

THE SLIMMER'S YEAR

Anne Ager · Julie Hamilton · Miriam Polunin

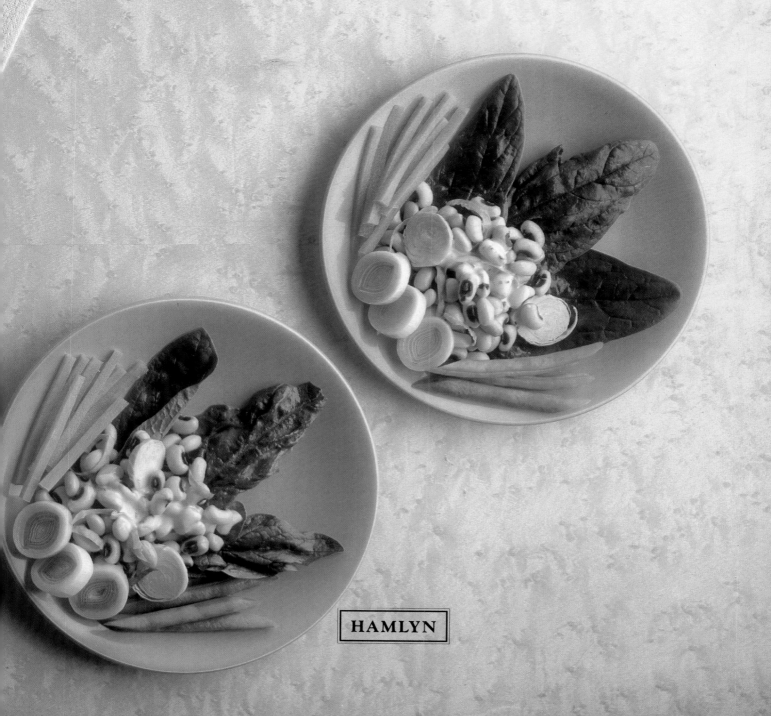

HAMLYN

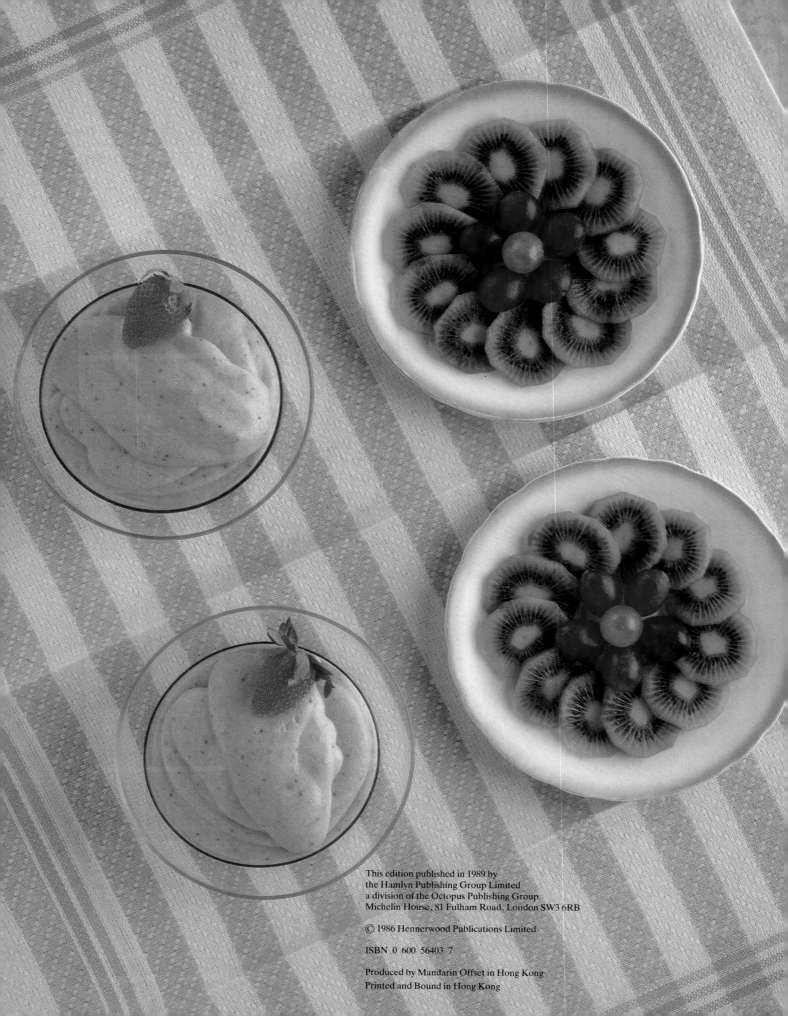

This edition published in 1989 by
the Hamlyn Publishing Group Limited
a division of the Octopus Publishing Group
Michelin House, 81 Fulham Road, London SW3 6RB

© 1986 Hennerwood Publications Limited

ISBN 0 600 56403 7

Produced by Mandarin Offset in Hong Kong
Printed and Bound in Hong Kong

CONTENTS

INTRODUCTION

Today there is a great interest in healthy eating. It is recognized that many of us are probably eating too much fat and sugar, possibly too much salt and not enough dietary fibre. For many people this type of diet, together with a sedentary lifestyle, has left them overweight and unfit. It has recently been estimated that about 32% of the female and 40% of the male population in Britain weigh more than is good for them. Some of these people are probably only marginally overweight but others have a real problem which is damaging their health, not only physically but mentally as well, because of the unhappiness it causes.

There is a joke about giving up smoking which could equally well be applied to slimming: 'Yes, giving up smoking (losing weight) is easy – I've done it dozens of times. . . .' Unfortunately, when applied to losing weight, this all too true. Many people 'go on a diet' once a week or once a month and keep to it for a few days or a week, only to slip up, eat something they feel they shouldn't and give up because they feel a failure once again.

Others may manage to keep to their diet for several months and succeed in losing all the excess weight, only to gradually regain the weight they lost once they return to a less restricted style of eating. Sadly, these 'long-term' dieters often find that they put the weight on again when seemingly eating less than they did before dieting. The reason for this is probably that their bodies have adapted to managing on less energy (food), and therefore treat even relatively small amounts of extra food as an excess energy supply and store it as fat.

With this in mind, ideas about slimming are changing from an emphasis on 'going on a diet' temporarily to the idea of permanently changing eating habits, with the aim of losing any excess weight slowly and of keeping it off. To succeed, this will mean finding a way of eating which does not make you feel deprived and which allows you to eat basically the same foods as everyone else. Even then you may not find the going easy because our eating habits have been firmly ingrained over a lifetime; it requires a great deal of determination and conscious thought, especially at first, to change them. The recipes in this book, however, are aimed at making the process easier, by providing tempting and imaginative, yet low

Calorie, menus for every sort of occasion, from quick family snacks to gourmet celebration dinners.

But first, some of the questions:

1. How much should I weigh?
It is difficult to assess anyone's ideal weight as everyone's individual build varies so much. Very often though, you can tell that you are overweight just by looking at yourself in a mirror; or because your clothes feel tighter than they once did. But for those who really want to know accurately, the charts opposite will enable you to estimate a suitable weight range according to your height. To find out how you rate:

1. Measure your height in bare feet.
2. Weigh yourself, preferably without clothes. If this is impossible remove your shoes and allow 2 kg (4–5 lb) for indoor clothes.
3. Find your height on the chart and draw a line across.
4. Find your weight and draw a line across here.
5. Mark where they cross, noting into what range it falls.

If it falls within the 'suitable' bracket, you are about right for your height. Weigh yourself occasionally to make sure you stay that way. If you are in the 'fat' category, you could probably benefit from losing some weight, so set yourself a target which is at the top of the 'suitable' range and reassess the situation when you get down to this. If you are in the 'very fat' section, your extra weight could be endangering your health. It has probably taken you a while to reach this weight and you should not underestimate the time it will take to reduce it. Set your initial target just inside the next range down and then think again when you reach this.

It is important to be realistic about the amount of weight that can be lost; even if you starved yourself you would only lose about 2.5 kg (5–6 lb) each week and you would be very unhealthy with it. Aim to lose about 1–2 lb per week. If you have not dieted before, or only for a while, you may lose more at first but this initial loss is mainly water and the rate will slow down later.

Just a word of warning: before attempting any weight reduction programme, it is advisable to check with your doctor.

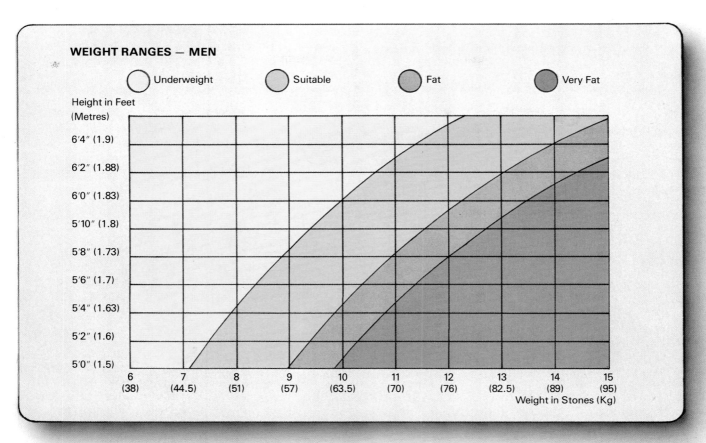

WEIGHT RANGES — MEN

Underweight   Suitable   Fat   Very Fat

Height in Feet (Metres)

6'4" (1.9)
6'2" (1.88)
6'0" (1.83)
5'10" (1.8)
5'8" (1.73)
5'6" (1.7)
5'4" (1.63)
5'2" (1.6)
5'0" (1.5)

6 (38)   7 (44.5)   8 (51)   9 (57)   10 (63.5)   11 (70)   12 (76)   13 (82.5)   14 (89)   15 (95)

Weight in Stones (Kg)

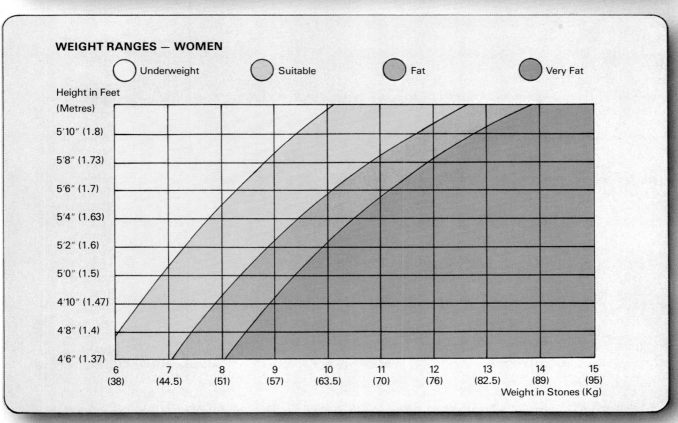

WEIGHT RANGES — WOMEN

Underweight   Suitable   Fat   Very Fat

Height in Feet (Metres)

5'10" (1.8)
5'8" (1.73)
5'6" (1.7)
5'4" (1.63)
5'2" (1.6)
5'0" (1.5)
4'10" (1.47)
4'8" (1.4)
4'6" (1.37)

6 (38)   7 (44.5)   8 (51)   9 (57)   10 (63.5)   11 (70)   12 (76)   13 (82.5)   14 (89)   15 (95)

Weight in Stones (Kg)

2. How many Calories?

In order to stay the same weight you have to balance the energy you take in as food with the energy you use up in living.

If you have gained weight you have been taking in more energy than you are using up and the excess has been stored as fat. In order to lose weight you need to use up some of this stored energy in your daily activities. So for a while, you need actually to take in less energy than you need.

Energy is still usually quoted in Calories, despite the scientists wanting us to use the proper term – Joules. One pound of fat has about 3500 Calories, so in order to lose one pound in weight you need to eat 3500 Calories fewer than the number you were eating to maintain your weight. Very few of us actually know how many Calories we eat from day to day, but one way to find out is to write down everything you eat for a week (see the Eating Diary on page 10). To get a realistic estimate, you need to be as accurate as possible about weights of portions and how foods are cooked. Then you should check the Calories against the charts in this book or one of the many lists available. If you want to lose about 1–2 lb each week you need to cut down on the total number of Calories consumed each week by about 3500–7000 Calories.

It might seem to be simpler to suggest cutting down by 500–1000 Calories every day. This arrangement is fine if you have a very regular lifestyle and a similar eating pattern each day of the week. For many people, however, it is more realistic to accept that our lives simply aren't organized like that, and it is wisest to calculate our Calorie intake on a weekly basis. Special celebrations, dinner parties or outings inevitably occur and extra food (or drink) will usually be consumed. On other days however perhaps you won't feel very hungry and will eat less anyway. Try to balance out the week's Calories between high days and low days but remaining within your weekly Calorie allowance. Remember you are trying to work out a way of eating to keep to permanently and it won't work unless it is flexible enough to fit into your lifestyle.

Do not reduce your energy intake below about 1200–1400 Calories each day, especially if you have a lot of weight to lose. You may lose weight faster but you may well fall into the trap of losing and gaining again.

3. What about exercise?

Since using up less energy than we eat means that we store it away as fat and gain weight, it would seem logical that an alternative method of losing weight would be to increase our level of exercise and use up some of the fat store. The chart opposite shows the amount of energy used by an adult weighing 70 kg (about 11 st) in the course of various activities. (A lighter person would use less and a heavier person more than this.) In fact, most people would need to do quite a lot of exercise in order to burn off a pound of fat (3500 Calories).

However, a great deal of interest has recently been shown in the possibility that regular sustained exercise may actually increase the rate at which the body metabolizes energy, even after you stop doing the exercise, and may therefore help you to lose weight. The exercise has to be 'aerobic', e.g. swimming, jogging, brisk walking or 'aerobic' exercises, all of which increase the supply of oxygen to the tissues. It must be done at a steady pace and increase your pulse-rate for 20–30 minutes at least 2–3 times each week. This is an exciting theory that is being investigated by nutritionists and physiologists. Exercise is also beneficial because it generates a feeling of relaxed well-being which means that over-eating due to tension is less likely, and there is some suggestion that it helps to control appetite. Exercise will also help to tone up flabby muscles and give you a sleeker outline.

Changing behaviour

Earlier it was emphasized that the ideal 'diet' is not a diet that is tried and then forgotten, but a pattern of eating which enables you to reach and maintain your own ideal weight and which you can make part of your life. This sounds relatively simple, but old patterns are not always easy to give up and, you may not really be aware of how much you eat or your reasons for doing so.

To become more aware of your own eating pattern it may help to keep a detailed record of your eating habits for a week or two. Don't just write down what you eat, but note also when, with whom, the mood you were in and how hungry you were. The chart on page 10 is an example of such a record. Look at your own chart critically and see if you can find any keys to why you have gained weight. For instance, do you eat if you are bored, or angry with someone, or when you are worried about something? If you can recognize this, perhaps you can think of a more direct way of dealing with these feelings, rather than eating. After all, you will still feel angry after you have eaten the bar of chocolate, and perhaps guilty as well!

Do you eat at particular times of the day, whether you are hungry or not, e.g. at lunchtime or as soon as you get home at night? If so, ask yourself if it is really necessary, and make a point of eating only if you are truly hungry. If you don't know what it is like to be hungry, be brave and try to postpone your meals until you are sure you know what hunger feels like.

A common reason for eating more than you really need at a meal is feeling generally harassed or short of time. Then, when you sit down to a meal you may swallow the food, hardly noticing it and certainly not enjoying it. Try to make time for yourself during the day, and allow yourself to relax before meals. This may actually enable you to enjoy your food and eat less.

Here are a few more ideas for changing your behaviour regarding food:

1. Enlist the help of those you live with; if you are tempted to eat when making snacks for others, persuade them to make their own. Ask them not to eat the foods which tempt you most in front of you; get them to congratulate you when you are successful at resisting temptation.

2. Serve yourself with smallish portions of food initially and don't leave the serving dishes on the table within

APPROXIMATE ENERGY COST OF SOME ACTIVITIES FOR A 70 KG ADULT

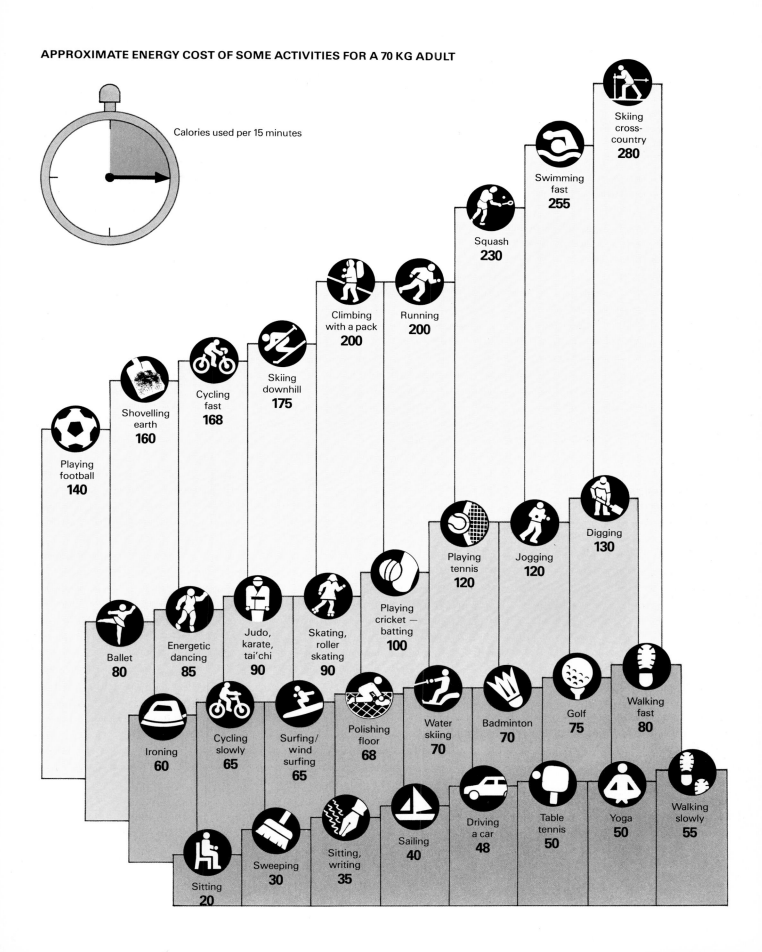

Calories used per 15 minutes

Skiing cross-country **280**

Swimming fast **255**

Squash **230**

Climbing with a pack **200**

Running **200**

Skiing downhill **175**

Cycling fast **168**

Shovelling earth **160**

Playing football **140**

Digging **130**

Jogging **120**

Playing tennis **120**

Playing cricket — batting **100**

Judo, karate, tai'chi **90**

Skating, roller skating **90**

Energetic dancing **85**

Ballet **80**

Walking fast **80**

Golf **75**

Water skiing **70**

Badminton **70**

Polishing floor **68**

Cycling slowly **65**

Surfing/wind surfing **65**

Ironing **60**

Walking slowly **55**

Yoga **50**

Table tennis **50**

Driving a car **48**

Sailing **40**

Sitting, writing **35**

Sweeping **30**

Sitting **20**

Eating Diary

TIME	PLACE	WITH WHOM	MOOD	HUNGRY	ACTIVITY BEFORE EATING	FOOD EATEN	ENERGY VALUE	DID I ENJOY IT
7·30	Kitchen	Alone	Sleepy	YES	Getting Up	Coffee (Black)		
						Branflakes (Bowl)	100	DON'T KNOW
						Milk	40	
						Orange Juice	50	YES
9·30	Office	Alone	Okay	NO	Opening Mail	Coffee (Black)		
						Chocolate Biscuits	130	YES
11·00	"	Colleagues	Harassed	NO	Working	Coffee (Black)		
						Two Biscuits	260	DIDN'T NOTICE
1·45	"	"	Okay	YES	Reading Paper	Cheese Sandwich	530	YES
						Apple	50	
						Coffee (Milky)	60	
5·30	Bus	Alone	Tired	YES	Walking to Bus Stop	Chocolate Bar	270	YES
6·15	Home Kitchen	Husband	Tired	MAYBE	Preparing Supper	2 Pieces of Carrot	10	DON'T KNOW
						Coffee (Milky)	60	
8·30	Dining Room	Husband + Friends	Cheerful	YES	Talking + Relaxing	Grilled Chop	560	YES
						Salad	30	
						Potatoes	120	BUT VERY
						Apple Pie	300	FULL
						Cream 1 tbsp	100	
						2 Glasses of white Wine	200	
						Coffee (Milky)	60	
						TOTAL	2930	

easy reach. You can have some more if you want it but you will have to go and get it.

3. Remember that you don't have to eat all the food on the plate, check with yourself during the meal to see if you have had enough. It is just as wasteful to eat food you don't need as it is to put it in the waste bin.

4. Eat slowly and taste each mouthful of food; you will begin to appreciate it more. Putting down your knife and fork between mouthfuls may help here.

5. To discourage any unnecessary nibbles make a chart recording your weight loss and stick it to the refrigerator door.

6. If you are following a recipe that uses only a small quantity of wine, and you have a little left over, rather than finish it up yourself, pour it into the freezer tray of your refrigerator, and freeze in cubes to use in recipes at a later date.

7. When you shop make a list of the foods you want to buy and keep to it. Go shopping when you have eaten, not when you are hungry.

8. Reward yourself whenever you resist temptation. Obviously, don't use food as a reward, but buy yourself a magazine or some flowers or allow yourself a long soak in the bath – anything that makes you feel good. Don't punish yourself when you feel you have 'gone wrong'; just accept it and forget it. If you let yourself feel guilty about it you will probably do it again sooner. Even if you follow these guidelines for healthy eating religiously, there are bound to be times when you eat something which is not ideal. There is nothing wrong with the occasional bar of chocolate or piece of cake if you are eating sensibly most of the time; it is only when you do it too often that the problems start.

A healthy eating pattern

The recipes in this book are designed to give you ideas for menus for each month of the year, using fresh foods when they are in season. They are also designed to fit with the ideas of a healthy diet, i.e. low in fat and salt, high in dietary fibre and with a good proportion of the energy being supplied by starchy carbohydrate ingredients like wholemeal cereals, potatoes and pulses.

Using these recipes will help you to develop a sensible way of eating but you need to make the rest of your diet conform to this pattern as well. Here are some ideas on how to do it:

Carbohydrate and dietary fibre

Your new eating pattern should be based on foods containing starchy carbohydrates with their dietary fibre intact. These foods will fill you up without giving you too many Calories, as dietary fibre is not broken down in the body to produce energy in the same way as sugars and starch. It therefore dilutes the energy in the food and may also prevent some of it from being absorbed into the body.

Current ideas suggest that we should eat at least 25–30 g of dietary fibre per day. So include at least three slices of wholemeal bread (about 10 g dietary fibre) in your daily Calorie allowance as well as some wholegrain cereal for breakfast. Pulses, such as lentils, dried peas and beans are another high fibre food: use these as a replacement for meat once or twice each week as they are also high in protein.

Vegetables and fruit supply useful amounts of dietary fibre and are filling. A meal based on fresh seasonal vegetables, with the meat, fish, eggs or cheese as a much less important part, is the basis of this new style of eating. Concentrate on fresh foods and avoid processed ones which can be high in fat and sugar.

Don't avoid potatoes; especially when baked in their jackets (eat the skin), they are another filling food. A medium baked potato (about 150 g/5 oz) would supply about 120 Calories. Other foods which make useful accompaniments to some of the recipes in this book, or can be useful as the basis of a meal, are brown rice (140 Calories per 100 g/4 oz cooked) and wholemeal pastas (120 Calories per 100 g/4 oz cooked weight).

Sugar and foods containing it don't come under the heading of healthy carbohydrate foods as all they provide is energy. So keep these to a minimum. Artificial sweeteners can be used to sweeten drinks if you have a sweet tooth and there are low-sugar jams and marmalades if you can't do without a little something on your toast in the morning. On the whole, though, it is better to wean yourself away from sweet foods.

Cutting down on fat
Some forms of fat like butter, margarines and oils are obvious, as is the visible fat on meat, and these should be limited. Don't fry foods unless you use a non-stick pan and no fat. Cut off visible fat from meat and choose the types low in fat like chicken or turkey. Have fish at least once a week. White fish is especially low in Calories.

There are also hidden sources of fat – cheese for example, is a high fat food (and also contains a lot of salt) and if you drink much milky tea or coffee you could be getting a good deal of energy from the milk. Low fat or skimmed milk is useful as it supplies all the protein and minerals of ordinary milk but is lower in fat and energy. Have 300 ml (½ pint) of skimmed milk or the equivalent in low fat yogurt each day to keep up your intake of the calcium needed for healthy bones. Low fat spreads have about half the Calories of butter and margarine and are a painless way of reducing your fat and energy intake. Experts believe we should get less than 35% of our energy supply from fat – so on 1500 Calories a day you will only need about 60 g of fat.

Avoiding salt
The foods which contain salt are generally processed foods, and include such things as bacon, ham and cheese as well as tinned meats and fish. The way to avoid having too much salt is therefore to keep to the basic principle of fresh foods as the main part of your diet. Use a very little salt in cooking vegetables or casseroles and don't add it at the table. Many people who have tried this have noticed that they appreciate the flavour of the food itself much more.

What not to do!
Don't try to lose weight by skipping meals, but divide your daily Calorie allowance up into at least three meals per day. There is a theory that it is better to have five or six small meals a day than one or two with a similar energy content, because each time you eat it perks up your metabolism and burns up more of the energy taken in. Whether or not this is so, eating little and often will prevent you from getting ravenously hungry and perhaps eating more than you intended.

It is often said that people should not miss breakfast, especially if they are trying to lose weight, but if you never eat breakfast then you might find it difficult to start now. On the other hand, if you are used to eating a big breakfast, possibly because you feel it is important to start the day well after a long time without food, you should think about whether you need that quantity of food. Some ideas for relatively low calorie breakfasts are:
– 2 tablespoons muesli with 65 ml (2½ fl oz) skimmed milk (230 Calories/960 kilojoules) or with 1 tablespoon yogurt (225 Calories/960 kilojoules)
– Half a grapefruit followed by 2 thin slices wholemeal toast with low fat spread and yeast extract (180 Calories/760 kilojoules)
– Small bowl of porridge plus 65 ml (2½ fl oz) skimmed milk (100 Calories/420 kilojoules)
– 1 boiled egg plus 1 slice of wholemeal bread or 2 crispbreads with low fat spread (160 Calories/670 kilojoules)
– 2 tablespoons bran cereal plus 100 ml (3½ fl oz) skimmed milk and fruit (e.g. ½ a peach) (160 Calories/670 kilojoules)

Eating out
It would be rather too much to expect you to have every meal at home when you develop this new way of eating. Eating in restaurants or in other people's homes can be full of pitfalls for anyone trying to watch what they eat, but these can be overcome. If you know you are going for a celebration meal, prepare for it by reducing your food intake a little over the preceding few days; then you can eat slightly more with a clear conscience. A word of warning though: it rarely works the other way round, i.e. promising you'll cut down for a few days after your celebration.

It is important to choose a restaurant where you can keep to your healthy eating pattern, i.e. where the menu includes food cooked without heavy sauces or lots of fat. Chinese food is often quite good but Indian meals are usually very high in fat. Simpler dishes, such as grilled meat and fish, are easier to find in Greek or Greek-Cypriot restaurants than in French or Italian restaurants.

To sum up, this book will help you develop a healthy eating pattern by giving you recipes for meals using the fresh, unprocessed foods that are available in each month of the year. Plan the rest of your diet around the guidelines given here, choosing your accompaniments to these recipes according to the tables here, that give you the energy, fat and dietary fibre content of the basic foods in season. Happy eating, and here's to a slimmer, and healthier year!

SPRING
March, April, May

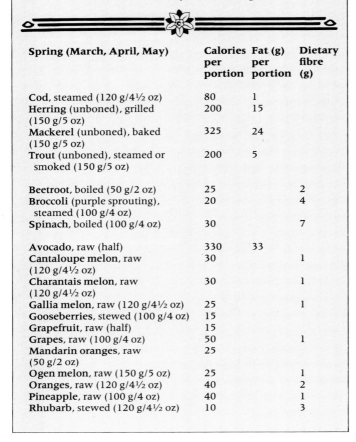

Spring (March, April, May)	Calories per portion	Fat (g) per portion	Dietary fibre (g)
Cod, steamed (120 g/4½ oz)	80	1	
Herring (unboned), grilled (150 g/5 oz)	200	15	
Mackerel (unboned), baked (150 g/5 oz)	325	24	
Trout (unboned), steamed or smoked (150 g/5 oz)	200	5	
Beetroot, boiled (50 g/2 oz)	25		2
Broccoli (purple sprouting), steamed (100 g/4 oz)	20		4
Spinach, boiled (100 g/4 oz)	30		7
Avocado, raw (half)	330	33	
Cantaloupe melon, raw (120 g/4½ oz)	30		1
Charantais melon, raw (120 g/4½ oz)	30		1
Gallia melon, raw (120 g/4½ oz)	25		1
Gooseberries, stewed (100 g/4 oz)	15		
Grapefruit, raw (half)	15		
Grapes, raw (100 g/4 oz)	50		1
Mandarin oranges, raw (50 g/2 oz)	25		
Ogen melon, raw (150 g/5 oz)	25		1
Oranges, raw (120 g/4½ oz)	40		2
Pineapple, raw (100 g/4 oz)	40		1
Rhubarb, stewed (120 g/4½ oz)	10		3

	Calories		Dietary fibre (g)
Broad beans, boiled (100 g/4 oz)	50		4
Broccoli (calabrese, green), steamed (100 g/4 oz)	20		4
Chinese leaves, raw (50 g/2 oz)	10		
Cos lettuce, raw (75 g/3 oz)	10		
Courgettes, steamed (100 g/4 oz)	10		
Cucumber, raw (25 g/1 oz)	5		
Endive, raw (50 g/2 oz)	10		
Fennel, steamed (50 g/2 oz)	15		1
French beans, steamed (100 g/4 oz)	10		3
Globe artichokes, boiled (1 medium)	10		
Lettuce, raw (50 g/2 oz)	5		1
New potatoes, steamed (120 g/4½ oz)	80		1
Garden peas, boiled (65 g/2½ oz)	25		3
Peppers, raw (50 g/2 oz)	10		
Radishes, raw (100 g/4 oz)	15		1
Runner beans, boiled (100 g/4 oz)	10		3
Spring onions, raw (25 g/1 oz)	5		3
Tomatoes, raw (100 g/4 oz)	15		2
Webbs lettuce, raw (50 g/2 oz)	5		1
Apricots, raw (100 g/4 oz)	25		2
Blackberries, raw (100 g/4 oz)	30		8
Black cherries, raw (100 g/4 oz)	40		2
Blackcurrants, raw (100 g/4 oz)	30		9
Gooseberries, raw (100 g/4 oz)	15		3
Grapes, raw (100 g/4 oz)	50		1
Loganberries, raw (100 g/4 oz)	15		6
Nectarines, raw (50 g/2 oz)	25		1
Peaches, raw (120 g/4½ oz)	40		1
Plums, raw (100 g/4 oz)	35		4
Raspberries, raw (100 g/4 oz)	25		
Red cherries, raw (100 g/4 oz)	40		2
Redcurrants, stewed (100 g/4 oz)	30		8
Strawberries, raw (100 g/4 oz)	25		2
Whitecurrants, stewed (100 g/4 oz)	30		8

SUMMER
June, July, August

Summer (June, July, August)	Calories per portion	Fat (g) per portion	Dietary fibre (g)
Lobster, boiled (120 g/4½ oz)	140	4	
Prawns, boiled (120 g/4½ oz)	130	1	
River trout (boned), steamed (150 g/5 oz)	200	7	
Salmon (boned), steamed (120 g/4½ oz)	240	15	
Sardines, grilled (65 g/2½ oz)	130	8	
Shrimps, boiled (65 g/2½ oz)	60	1	
Asparagus, boiled (100 g/4 oz)	10		1
Aubergine, steamed (100 g/4 oz)	15		3

AUTUMN
September, October, November

Autumn (September, October, November)	Calories per portion	Fat (g) per portion	Dietary fibre (g)
Mussels, boiled (120 g/4½ oz)	80	3	
Pheasant, roast (100 g/4 oz)	210	6	
Partridge, roast (100 g/4 oz)	210	7	
Scallops, steamed (100 g/4 oz)	100	1	
Wild duck, roast (100 g/4 oz)	190	10	
Celery, raw (50 g/2 oz)	5		1
Corn on the cob, boiled (150 g/5 oz)	190		3
Jerusalem artichokes, boiled (50 g/2 oz)	10		
Marrow, steamed (100 g/4 oz)	10		

Apples (eating), raw (120 g/4½ oz)	45	2
Apples (cooking), stewed (100 g/4 oz)	35	2
Blackberries, raw (100 g/4 oz)	30	8
Clementines, raw (50 g/2oz, unskinned weight)	20	1
Damsons, raw (100 g/4 oz)	35	4
Greengages, raw (100 g/4 oz)	45	3
Passion fruit, raw (25 g/1 oz)	15	2
Pears, raw (120 g/4½ oz)	40	2
Plums, raw (100 g/4 oz)	35	4
Quinces, stewed (100 g/4 oz)	25	7
Satsuma, raw (50 g/2oz, unskinned weight)	20	1
Tangerines, raw (50 g/2oz, unskinned weight)	20	1

WINTER
December, January, February

Winter (December, January, February)	Calories per portion	Fat (g) per portion	Dietary fibre (g)
Duck, roast (no skin) (100 g/4 oz)	190	10	
Finnan Haddie, poached (150 g/5 oz)	150	2	
Haddock, steamed (150 g/5 oz)	150	2	
Halibut, steamed (150 g/5 oz)	150	4	
Herrings, grilled (150 g/5 oz)	280	20	
Lemon sole, grilled (120 g/4½ oz)	110	1	
Pheasant, roast (100 g/4 oz)	200	10	
Plaice, steamed (120 g/4½ oz)	110	2	
Rabbit, roast (120 g/4½ oz)	220	10	
Smoked mackerel, grilled (100 g/4 oz)	290	16	
Turkey, roast (no skin) (100 g/4 oz)	110	4	
Brussels sprouts, steamed (100 g/4 oz)	20		3
Celeriac, boiled (100 g/4 oz)	15		3
Leeks, steamed (100 g/4 oz)	25		4
Parsnips, boiled (120 g/4½ oz)	70		3
Red cabbage, raw (50 g/2 oz)	10		2
Swede, boiled (120 g/4½ oz)	20		4
Sweet potatoes, boiled (100 g/4 oz)	85		3
Turnips, boiled (150 g/5 oz)	20		3
White cabbage, raw (50 g/2 oz)	10		2
Apricots, raw (100 g/4 oz)	25		2
Apples (Cox's), raw (120 g/4½ oz)	45		2
Cranberries, stewed (50 g/2 oz)	10		2
Dates (fresh), raw (50 g/2 oz)	80		3
Figs (fresh), raw (100 g/4 oz)	40		3
Honeydew melon (100 g/4 oz)	25		1
Lychees, raw (100 g/4 oz)	70		1
Orange, raw (120 g/4½ oz)	40		2
Rhubarb, raw (100 g/4 oz)	10		3

ALL YEAR ROUND

ALL YEAR ROUND	Calories per portion	Fat (g) per portion	Dietary fibre (g)
Beef, roast (100 g/4 oz)	190	27	
Chicken breasts, no skin, roast (100 g/4 oz)	140	14	
Crab (100 g/4 oz)	80	1	
Lamb, roast, lean (100 g/4 oz)	190	8	
Monkfish, steamed (100 g/4 oz)	100	1	
Pork, roast, lean (100 g/4 oz)	200	11	
Poussin, roast (150 g/5oz, unboned)	150	5	
Smoked ham (50 g/2 oz)	85	3	
Streaky bacon, grilled (1 rasher, 40 g/1½ oz)	170	14	
Veal, roast (100 g/4 oz)	230	12	
Black-eyed beans, cooked (100 g/4 oz)	95	1	8
Chick peas, cooked (100 g/4 oz)	140	3	6
Lentils, cooked (100 g/4 oz)	100	1	4
Kidney beans, canned (100 g/4 oz)	95	1	8
Eggs (50 g/2 oz, 1 egg)	80	10	
Low fat spread (10 g/¼ oz)	35	4	
Skimmed milk (300ml/½ pint)	100		
Olive oil (25 g/1 oz)	300	30	
Whole milk (300ml/½ pint)	200	12	
Yogurt, plain, unsweetened (150 g/5oz, small carton)	75	2	
Cottage cheese (25 g/1 oz)	25	1	
Cream cheese (25 g/1 oz)	110	12	
Edam cheese (25 g/1 oz)	75	6	
Parmesan cheese (25 g/1 oz)	40	3	
Petit Suisse (25 g/1 oz)	100	7	
Cheddar cheese (25 g/1 oz)	120	10	
Brown rice, cooked (100 g/4 oz)	120		2
Bulgar wheat, raw (50 g/2 oz)	175		4
Muesli (65 g/2½ oz)	220	4	4
Pitta bread, white (100 g/4 oz)	260	2	3
Pumpernickel bread (50 g/2 oz)	120	1	
Rye bread (100 g/4 oz)	240	1	
Wholemeal bread and rolls (100 g/4 oz)	220	3	9
Potatoes, baked with skin (200 g/7 oz)	170		4
Bean sprouts, raw (50 g/2 oz)	5		2
Carrots, raw (50 g/2 oz)	10		2
Cauliflower, steamed (100 g/4 oz)	10		2
Green cabbage, steamed (100 g/4 oz)	10		3
Mushrooms, raw (25 g/1 oz)	5		1
Onions (peeled), raw (100 g/4 oz)	25		1
Round lettuce, raw (50 g/2 oz)	5		1
Spring greens, boiled (50 g/2 oz)	5		2
Bananas (120 g/4½ oz)	95		5
Lemons (100 g/4 oz)	15		5
Mango (100 g/4 oz)	60		2
Raisins (20 g/¾ oz)	50		2
Sultanas (20 g/¾ oz)	50		2

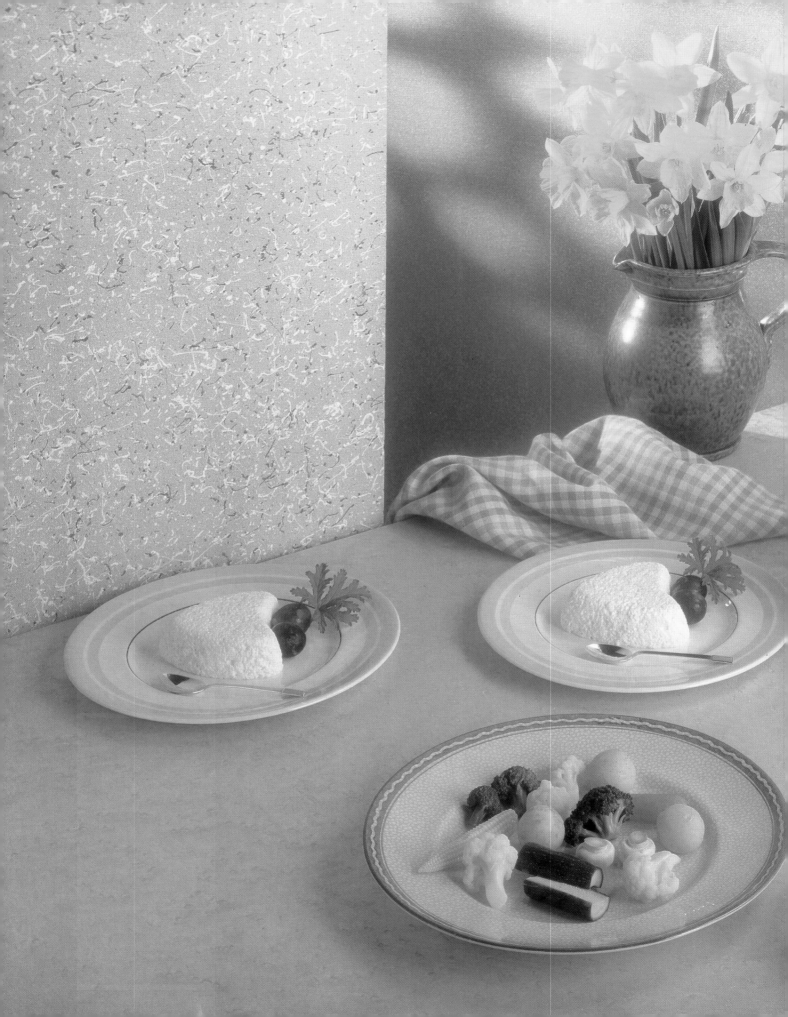

SPRING

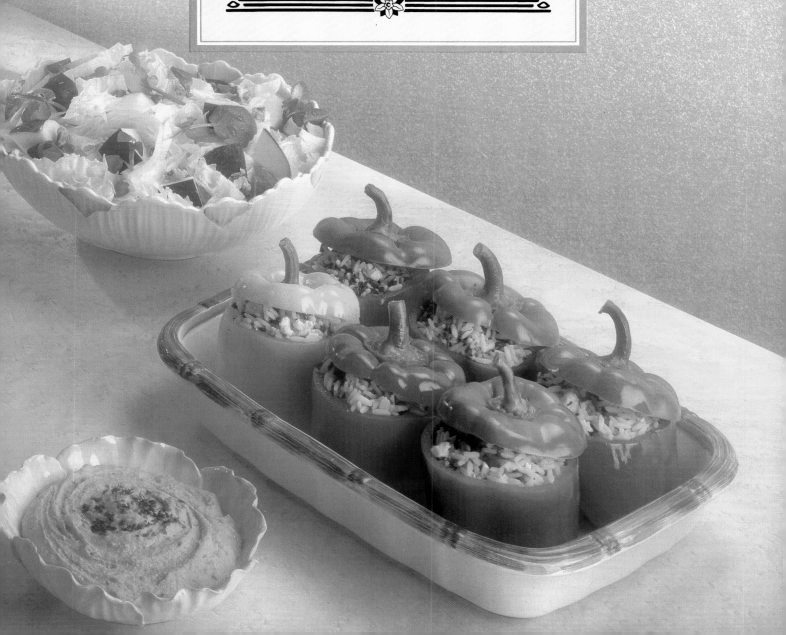

MARCH

Shrove Tuesday Pancake Party for Eight

Shrove Tuesday is an excuse to hold a delightfully informal party, making pancakes the centre-piece. Even though it does not fall on the same date each year, and may occur in February if Easter is early, it always seems to be a herald of spring.

Marinated Mushrooms

450 g (1 lb) small button
  mushrooms, wiped
1 teaspoon salt
1 tablespoon oil
1 tablespoon lemon juice
2 tablespoons white wine
  vinegar
1 teaspoon sugar

PREPARATION TIME:
15 minutes, plus marinating
COOKING TIME:
10 minutes
CALORIES PER PORTION:
25 (105 kilojoules)

1. Boil the mushrooms in a large pan of lightly salted water for 1 minute, then drain, reserving 3 tablespoons of water.
2. Combine the oil with the lemon juice, vinegar and reserved mushroom water and add the sugar and mushrooms. Bring to the boil, remove from the heat at once and leave to cool uncovered. Marinate for at least 12 hours.
3. Serve in the liquid.

Pancakes Stuffed with Ricotta Cheese and Spinach

Pancake batter:
300 ml (10 fl oz) skimmed
  milk
250 ml (8 fl oz) soda water
pinch of salt
2 eggs
225 g (8 oz) strong white
  plain flour, sifted
15 g (1/2 oz) butter
Filling:
225 g (8 oz) fresh spinach
400 g (14 oz) Ricotta cheese
1 egg (size 1), lightly beaten
1/2 teaspoon grated lemon rind
1/2 teaspoon ground cinnamon
1/2 teaspoon salt
freshly ground black pepper
1 tablespoon chopped fresh
  chives, to garnish

PREPARATION TIME:
20–30 minutes, plus resting
COOKING TIME:
about 1 hour
OVEN TEMPERATURE:
180°C, 350°F, Gas Mark 4
CALORIES PER PORTION:
290 (1220 kilojoules)

1. Combine the milk, soda water and salt in a jug. Combine the eggs and flour in a large bowl and beat vigorously, adding the milk and water mixture at the same time. Beat until you have a smooth creamy texture and set aside for 30 minutes to thicken.
2. Smear an 18 cm (7 inch) heavy-based shallow frying pan with just enough butter to gloss the surface. Place over a fierce heat and when the pan is very hot pour in 1/16 of the batter tilting the pan to spread it. Cook for 1 minute until golden, then flip the pancake with a palette knife or spatula and cook the other side for 1 minute. Remove. Cook 15 more pancakes in the same way.
3. Wash and trim the spinach, then wring it out very thoroughly as you would a dishcloth, squeezing out as much of the liquid as you can, then chop it and mix it with the Ricotta cheese. Add the egg, lemon rind, cinnamon, salt and pepper and mix thoroughly.
4. Spread the mixture over each pancake, roll up and place, seam down, side by side in a shallow ovenproof dish. Cover lightly with buttered greaseproof paper and bake in a preheated oven for about 20 minutes.
5. Garnish with chives just before serving.

CLOCKWISE FROM TOP LEFT
Marinated mushrooms; Apple and walnut salad; Pancakes stuffed with Ricotta cheese and spinach; Avocado, lime and melon dessert salad

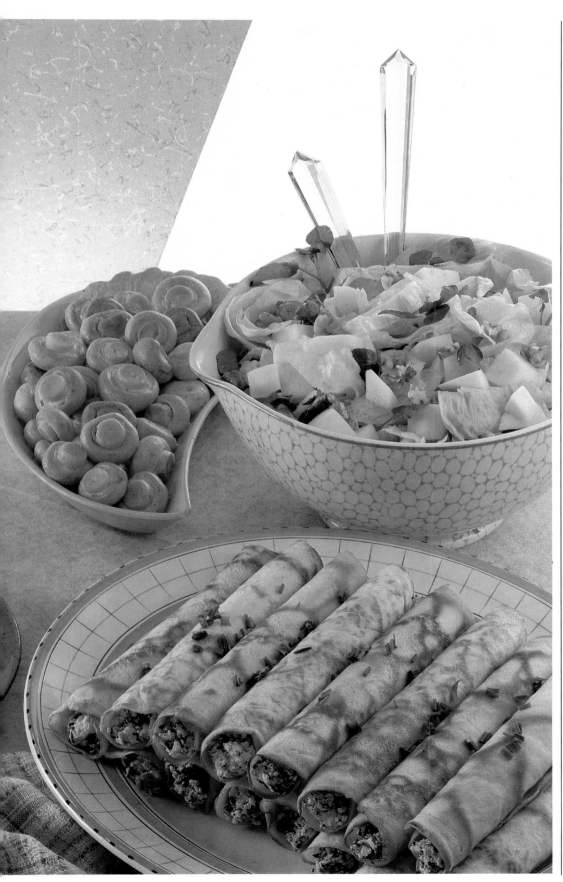

Apple and Walnut Salad

1 iceberg lettuce, sliced
2 bunches watercress,
  trimmed and chopped
1 apple, peeled, cubed and
  tossed in lemon juice
50 g (2 oz) walnuts, chopped
1 tablespoon walnut oil
2 tablespoons wine vinegar
salt
freshly ground black pepper

PREPARATION TIME:
10 minutes
CALORIES PER PORTION:
70 (290 kilojoules)

1. Mix the lettuce with the watercress and apple.
2. Sprinkle the walnuts over and drizzle on the walnut oil and vinegar. Season with salt and pepper. Toss the salad before serving.

Avocado, Lime and Melon Dessert Salad

1 large honeydew melon
2 medium avocado pears
1 tablespoon Kirsch (optional)
juice of 3 limes
lime slices, to garnish

PREPARATION TIME:
15–20 minutes
CALORIES PER PORTION:
110 (460 kilojoules)

1. Quarter the melons and remove the pips. Cut off the skin, then cut the flesh into thin widthways slices.
2. Halve, stone and peel the avocados and slice them lengthways. Arrange the fruit on 8 dessert plates. Combine the Kirsch and lime juice and pour over. Cover tightly with cling film until ready to serve. Do not chill.
3. Garnish each plate with 2 lime slices before serving.

MARCH

Hors d'oeuvres and Light Meals

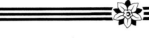

Poached Eggs with Anchovy Sauce

4 tablespoons plain unsweetened yogurt
1 tablespoon low calorie mayonnaise
2 teaspoons anchovy essence
1 teaspoon finely grated lemon rind
freshly ground black pepper
4 thin slices wholemeal bread
15 g (½ oz) low fat spread
1 tablespoon sesame seeds
¼ teaspoon salt
2 teaspoons white wine vinegar
4 eggs

PREPARATION TIME:
15 minutes
COOKING TIME:
4–5 minutes
CALORIES PER PORTION:
140 (590 kilojoules)

An unusual and piquant adaptation of a well-known dish. The eggs can be served as a light weekday lunch, as a special weekend breakfast treat, or as a starter to an informal supper.

1. Mix the yogurt with the mayonnaise, anchovy essence, lemon rind and pepper to taste.
2. Spread the slices of wholemeal bread very thinly with low fat spread; sprinkle with sesame seeds.
3. Half fill a deep frying pan with water; add the salt and vinegar and bring just to the boil.
4. Crack the eggs carefully, so that the yolks do not break, and lower them one by one into the gently bubbling water; poach for 2–3 minutes, spooning the fluffy white up and over the yolks as the eggs cook.
5. While the eggs are cooking, put the slices of sesame-topped bread under a preheated grill until lightly golden.
6. Drain the poached eggs carefully on a perforated slice and place one on each slice of sesame toast. Spoon the prepared anchovy sauce over the top, and serve immediately.

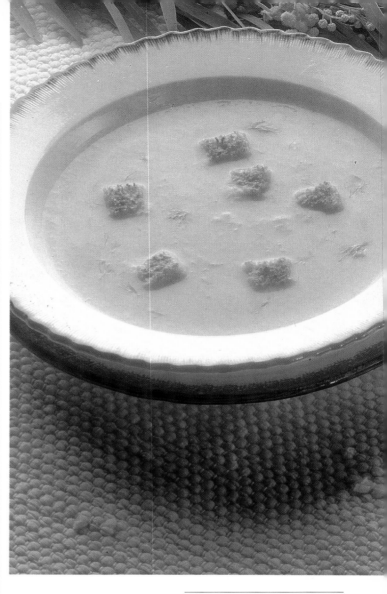

Aubergine Omelette with Celery and Orange Salad

1 large aubergine, thinly sliced
salt
6 celery sticks, cut into matchstick strips
3 oranges, peeled and divided into segments
1 tablespoon chopped fresh mint
4 tablespoons orange juice
freshly ground black pepper
6 eggs
2 tablespoons chopped fresh parsley
1 garlic clove, peeled and crushed
100 g (4 oz) Mozzarella cheese, cut into thin slivers

PREPARATION TIME:
45 minutes, plus draining
COOKING TIME:
about 15 minutes
OVEN TEMPERATURE:
190°C, 375°F, Gas Mark 5
CALORIES PER PORTION:
300 (1800 kilojoules)

1. Put the aubergine slices into a colander and sprinkle generously with salt. Leave to drain for 30 minutes, then rinse and pat dry with paper towels. Steam the slices over hot water for 3 minutes.
2. Mix the celery strips, orange segments and chopped mint together in a bowl. Spoon over the orange juice and season with salt and pepper to taste; toss lightly together.
3. Beat the eggs with 1 tablespoon water, the

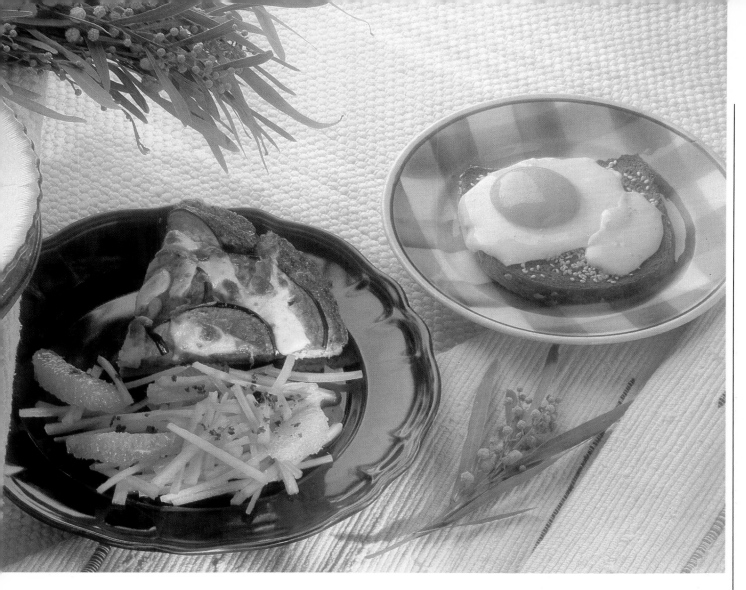

chopped parsley, garlic and salt and pepper to taste.
4. Pour the egg mixture into a non-stick frying pan and stir over a gentle heat, drawing the set egg mixture into the centre of the pan as it cooks.
5. Once the underside of the omelette is set, remove the pan from the heat. Arrange the aubergine slices overlapping on the top and sprinkle with the thin slivers of Mozzarella cheese. Pop the omelette under a preheated grill until the cheese melts.
6. Serve piping hot, cut into wedges, with the celery and orange salad.

Fennel Soup

2 medium heads fennel, with leaves
1 medium onion, peeled and finely chopped
600 ml (1 pint) chicken stock
150 ml (¼ pint) skimmed milk
salt
freshly ground black pepper
1 teaspoon Pesto sauce
small wholemeal croûtons, to serve

PREPARATION TIME:
5 minutes
COOKING TIME:
20 minutes
CALORIES PER PORTION:
175 (730 kilojoules)

Jars of pesto sauce can be bought from Italian delicatessens and good supermarkets.

1. Remove the feathery leaves from the fennel, and keep them somewhere cool to use as a garnish. Trim any discoloured patches from the fennel, then shred both heads.
2. Put the shredded fennel into a pan with the onion, chicken stock, skimmed milk and salt and pepper to taste. Bring to the boil and simmer gently for about 20 minutes until the fennel is just tender.
3. Blend the soup in the liquidizer until smooth. Return to a clean saucepan, add the Pesto sauce and heat through.
4. Ladle the hot soup into small bowls. Garnish with fennel leaves, and serve with wholemeal croûtons.

FROM THE LEFT Fennel soup; Aubergine omelette with celery and orange salad; Poached eggs with anchovy sauce

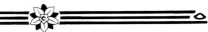

MARCH

Main Courses

Lemon Chicken

1 lemon, very thinly peeled, rind reserved
1 small onion, thinly sliced
2 tablespoons olive oil
4 skinned and boned chicken breasts, 150 g (5 oz) each
2 tablespoons chopped parsley
300 ml (½ pint) chicken stock
1 tablespoon clear honey
salt
freshly ground black pepper
2 teaspoons cornflour
1 tablespoon water

PREPARATION TIME:
15 minutes
COOKING TIME:
30–35 minutes
CALORIES PER PORTION:
320 (1330 kilojoules)

1. Cut the lemon rind into matchstick strips. Halve the lemon and squeeze out the juice.
2. Fry the onion gently in the oil for 3–4 minutes, then add the chicken breasts and fry until lightly browned on all sides.
3. Add the parsley, stock, honey, salt and pepper to taste and lemon juice; cover the pan and simmer gently for 20 minutes.
4. Remove the chicken breasts to a warmed serving dish, and keep warm.
5. Blend the cornflour and water to a smooth paste; stir in the hot cooking liquid, and then return to the pan. Stir over a gentle heat until thickened.
6. Add the strips of rind to the sauce and spoon evenly over the chicken.

Spaghetti with Three Herbs Sauce

3 tablespoons chopped fresh parsley
1 tablespoon chopped fresh tarragon
2 tablespoons chopped fresh basil
1 tablespoon olive oil
1 large garlic clove, peeled and crushed
4 tablespoons chicken stock
2 tablespoons dry white wine
salt
freshly ground black pepper
350 g (12 oz) wholewheat spaghetti

PREPARATION TIME:
15 minutes
COOKING TIME:
about 12 minutes
CALORIES PER PORTION:
325 (1370 kilojoules)

1. Put the parsley, tarragon, basil, olive oil, garlic, chicken stock, white wine and salt and pepper to taste into the liquidizer; blend until smooth.
2. Cook the spaghetti in a large pan of boiling salted water until just tender; test a strand from time to time, as wholewheat spaghetti takes longer to cook than the standard variety (about 12 minutes in total).
3. Drain the spaghetti and heap in a warmed bowl; pour over the herb sauce and toss well.

FROM THE LEFT Spaghetti with three herbs sauce; Lamb cutlets provençal; Lemon chicken

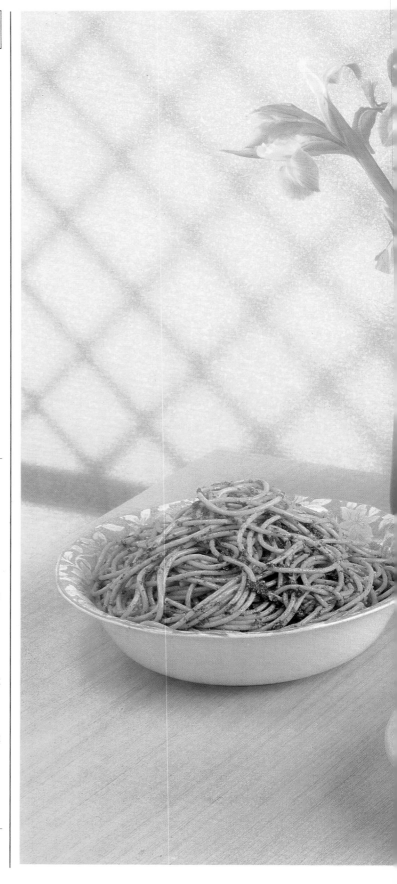

Lamb Cutlets Provençal

8 trimmed lamb cutlets
½ tablespoon olive oil
3 tablespoons red wine
salt
freshly ground black pepper
1 tablespoon chopped fresh
* basil*
1 red pepper, seeded and
* chopped*
6 tomatoes, skinned, seeded
* and chopped*
4 courgettes, chopped
1 small onion, peeled and
* finely chopped*
300 ml (½ pint) chicken stock
1 garlic clove, peeled and
* crushed*
1 tablespoon tomato purée
fresh basil, to garnish

PREPARATION TIME:
30–35 minutes, plus chilling
COOKING TIME:
10–12 minutes
CALORIES PER PORTION:
305 (1290 kilojoules)

1. Put the lamb cutlets into a shallow dish with the olive oil, wine, salt and pepper to taste and the chopped basil; cover and chill for 4 hours.
2. Put the red pepper, tomatoes, courgettes and onion into a pan with the chicken stock, garlic, tomato purée and salt and pepper to taste; simmer gently until the vegetables are just tender.
3. Drain the marinade from the lamb cutlets; blend the marinade and vegetable sauce in a liquidizer until smooth.
4. Cook the lamb cutlets under a preheated grill for 2–3 minutes on each side. Heat the sauce through.
5. Spoon a pool of vegetable sauce on to 4 plates and carefully arrange 2 cutlets on top of each.
6. Garnish with sprigs of basil and serve.

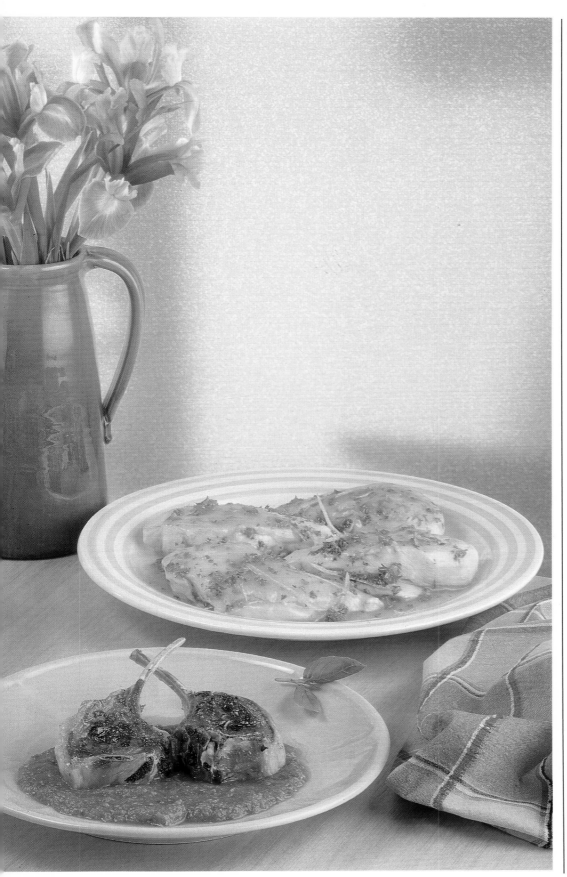

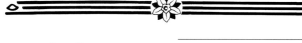

MARCH

Puddings

Poached Oranges with Raisins

4 large oranges
300 ml (½ pint) dry white
  wine
50 g (2 oz) raisins
1 teaspoon powdered gelatine
2 tablespoons dry vermouth

PREPARATION TIME:
25 minutes, plus cooling
COOKING TIME:
14 minutes
CALORIES PER PORTION:
155 (650 kilojoules)

1. Pare the rind from the oranges very thinly and cut it into fine matchstick strips. Put these into a pan with sufficient water to cover; bring to the boil and simmer for 4 minutes.

Drain thoroughly and plunge the strips into a bowl of iced water.
2. Remove all the pith from the peeled oranges; remove stubborn pieces with a clean razor blade.
3. Put the oranges into a pan with the wine and raisins; simmer gently for 10 minutes, turning the oranges from time to time.
4. Remove the oranges with a slotted spoon and place in a serving dish.
5. Dissolve the gelatine in the vermouth and stir into the cooking liquid; allow to cool and add half the orange rind strips. Spoon over the whole oranges, and scatter the remaining strips of rind around the oranges. Leave until completely cold.

Iced Grapefruit and Melon

4 grapefruit
artificial sweetener, to taste
1 small ripe melon
sprigs of fresh mint, to
  decorate

PREPARATION TIME:
30 minutes, plus chilling
CALORIES PER PORTION:
40 (170 kilojoules)

1. Trim all the pith and peel from the grapefruit; holding the fruit over a bowl, cut into the centre of each fruit on either side of each segment membrane, to separate the segments. (Catch as much juice as you can in the bowl.)
2. Add artificial sweetener

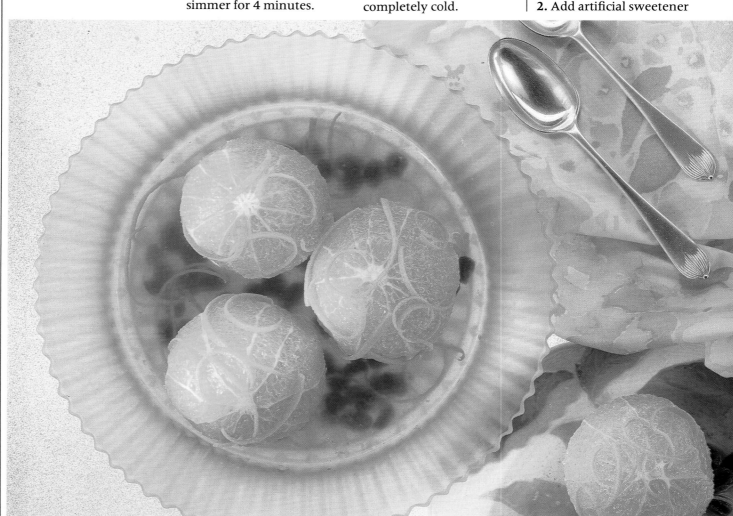

to taste to the juice; stir in the grapefruit segments.

3. Halve the melon and scoop out the seeds; using a melon ball cutter, cut the flesh into small balls.

4. Add the melon balls to the grapefruit segments, and mix together in the juice. Cover and chill for 1–2 hours.

5. Spoon the melon balls and grapefruit segments into small sundae dishes and decorate with sprigs of mint.

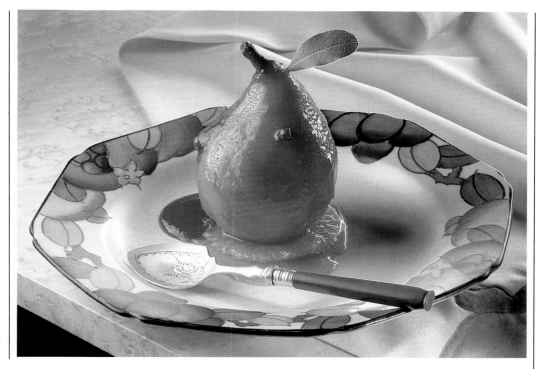

RIGHT Spiced pears

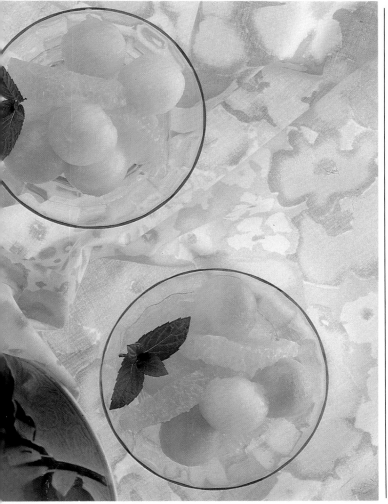

Spiced Pears

4 large firm pears
½ lemon
16 cloves
½ cinnamon stick
300 ml (½ pint) red wine
2 tablespoons redcurrant jelly
4 orange slices
4 small fresh bay leaves, to
* decorate*

PREPARATION TIME:
20 minutes
COOKING TIME:
about 16 minutes
CALORIES PER PORTION:
140 (590 kilojoules)

1. Peel the pears, leaving the stalks intact; rub them all over with the lemon half to prevent discoloration.

2. Stud each pear with 4 cloves. Stand them upright in a pan; add the cinnamon stick, wine and sufficient water just to cover the pears.

3. Bring to the boil and simmer gently until the pears are just tender. Leave to cool in the cooking liquid.

4. Put 2 tablespoons of the cooking liquid into a small pan with the redcurrant jelly; bubble briskly for about 1 minute until the jelly has dissolved.

5. Place an orange slice on each of 4 small plates; drain the pears with a slotted spoon, and sit one on top of each orange slice.

6. Spoon a little redcurrant glaze over each pear and decorate with a small bay leaf.

FROM THE LEFT Poached oranges with raisins; Iced grapefruit and melon

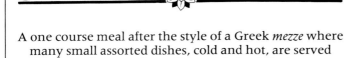

MARCH

Dinner Party for Six

A one course meal after the style of a Greek *mezze* where many small assorted dishes, cold and hot, are served simultaneously. Follow with fresh fruit.

Stuffed Spinach Leaves

100 g (4 oz) fresh haddock, boned and skinned
175 g (6 oz) crabmeat
1 egg white (size 1)
1 tablespoon lemon juice plus 1 teaspoon
1 teaspoon anchovy essence
freshly ground black pepper
salt
1 teaspoon olive oil
25 g (1 oz) long-grain rice
50 ml (2 fl oz) water
18 undamaged spinach, cabbage or vine leaves
1 tablespoon whipping cream

PREPARATION TIME:
50 minutes, plus chilling and standing
COOKING TIME:
55–60 minutes
OVEN TEMPERATURE:
180°C, 350°F, Gas Mark 4
CALORIES PER PORTION:
100 (420 kilojoules)

1. Place the haddock in a food processor with the crabmeat, egg white, 1 teaspoon lemon juice and anchovy essence and blend until smooth. Taste and add pepper and a little salt if necessary. Chill the mixture for 30 minutes.
2. Gently heat the oil in a saucepan, add the rice and toss until thoroughly coated. Add the water and simmer uncovered until it has been absorbed. Remove from the heat and leave to cool. The rice will only be partially cooked.
3. Wash the spinach, trim the stalks back to the leafy parts and place in a large bowl; pour boiling water over to cover and leave to stand for 3–4 minutes. Drain and dry thoroughly with paper towels.
4. Lightly whip the cream and combine it with the fish mixture, folding in the partially cooked rice at the same time.
5. Place a dollop of the mixture on a spinach leaf, fold in the sides and, starting with the stalk end, roll the leaf up to form a compact parcel. Prepare the rest of the spinach leaves in the same way. Pack the stuffed leaves into a greased gratin dish, pour over the tablespoon of lemon juice mixed with a tablespoon of water and cover. Place in a roasting tin half-filled with water and bake in a preheated oven for about 1 hour. Allow to cool completely, with the lid on.
6. To serve, arrange the parcels on a platter.

Individual Parmigianas

750 g (1½ lb) aubergines
3 eggs, beaten
salt
freshly ground black pepper
flour, for coating
1 dessertspoon oil
1 × 500 g (1 lb 2 oz) can tomatoes
1 tablespoon chopped fresh basil
150 g (5 oz) Ricotta cheese
100 g (4 oz) grated Parmesan cheese

PREPARATION TIME:
15 minutes
COOKING TIME:
about 1 hour
OVEN TEMPERATURE:
190°C, 375°F, Gas Mark 5
CALORIES PER PORTION:
220 (930 kilojoules)

1. Peel the aubergines and cut them lengthways into 5 mm (¼ inch) thick slices. Season the beaten eggs with salt and pepper. Dredge the aubergine slices in flour and dip them in the beaten egg.
2. Brush a griddle pan or non-stick frying pan with the oil for frying, add the aubergines and fry until golden, then drain on paper towels and set aside.
3. Sieve the tomatoes.
4. Put the tomatoes and basil in a saucepan, bring to the boil and simmer until reduced by about half; season lightly.
5. Cover the bottom of 6 individual ovenproof dishes with a layer of aubergine, then dot with Ricotta cheese, cover with a layer of the tomato sauce and sprinkle a little Parmesan over. Repeat the process, ending with a layer of aubergine topped only by tomato and Parmesan.
6. Bake in a preheated oven for about 15 minutes.

Broccoli Dressed with Nutmeg and Lemon

1 kg (2 lb) fresh broccoli
1 teaspoon olive oil
2 very thin strips of lemon rind, about 4 cm (1½ inches) long
2 tablespoons lemon juice
generous pinch of grated nutmeg
salt
freshly ground black pepper

PREPARATION TIME:
10 minutes
COOKING TIME:
10 minutes, plus standing
CALORIES PER PORTION:
45 (190 kilojoules)

1. Trim most of the stalk off the broccoli heads. Peel the stalks and slice them thinly, diagonally. Wash the heads and break into small florets.
2. Steam the broccoli heads for 8 minutes, then taste to see if they are done; they should still have some bite.
3. While the heads are steaming, cook the stalks. Heat the oil in a wok or large frying pan until very hot, add the lemon rind and fry it until it starts to brown, then quickly add the sliced stalks. Stir-fry for barely 1 minute, then add the lemon juice, nutmeg and salt and pepper and fry for a further 30 seconds.
4. Place the steamed florets in a serving dish and lay stalks on top. Stir once then leave to cool.
5. Serve while still tepid.

CLOCKWISE FROM TOP Broccoli dressed with nutmeg and lemon; Terracotta baked potatoes; Grilled and marinated fresh sardines; Individual parmigianas CENTRE Stuffed spinach leaves

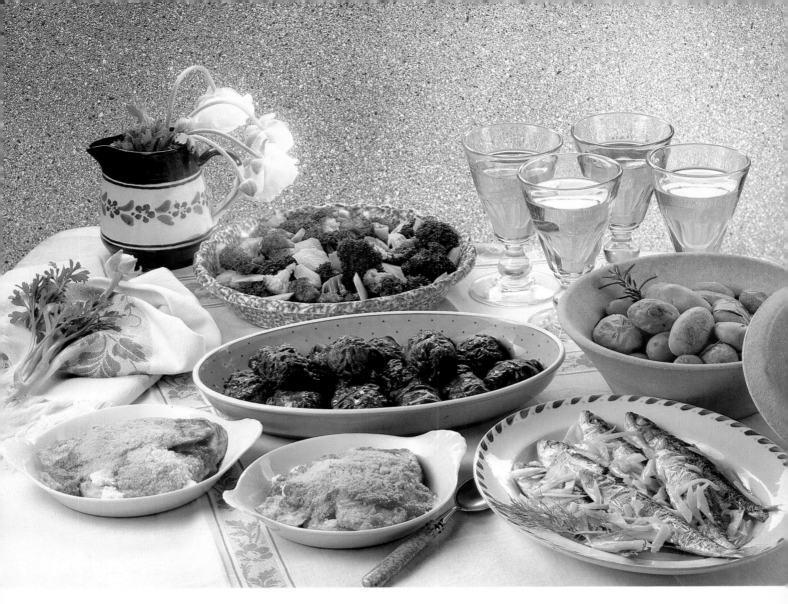

Terracotta Baked Potatoes

750 g (1½ lb) small new
  potatoes (approximately 24)
2 sprigs fresh rosemary
1 tablespoon lemon juice
1 tablespoon water
½ teaspoon salt

PREPARATION TIME:
10 minutes
COOKING TIME:
60 minutes
OVEN TEMPERATURE:
220°C, 425°F, Gas Mark 7
CALORIES PER PORTION:
100 (420 kilojoules)

This way of cooking
potatoes is really only
practical in an
earthenware or terracotta
casserole with a lid.

1. Wash the potatoes
carefully, trying not to
damage the skin which
must remain on, and place
them in a casserole.
2. Strip the rosemary
needles off the sprigs and
add them to the potatoes.
Sprinkle the lemon juice,
water and salt over, put
the lid on and shake the
pot well.
3. Place in a preheated
oven and bake for 60
minutes. Test the potatoes
at the end of the cooking
time, they may need a few
minutes more. Serve hot.

Grilled and Marinated Fresh Sardines

6 large sardines
salt
2 teaspoons olive oil
1 garlic clove, peeled and
  chopped
½ fennel bulb, finely sliced,
  leaves reserved
2 tablespoons wine vinegar
4 tablespoons white wine

PREPARATION TIME:
20 minutes, plus 2 days marinating
COOKING TIME:
30 minutes
CALORIES PER PORTION:
100 (420 kilojoules)

1. Wash the sardines,
removing the heads if
preferred. Carefully slit the
stomach of each sardine
and remove the innards.
2. Thoroughly dry the fish
and grill them under a
medium heat until crisp
and lightly browned.
Arrange them in a shallow
earthenware or terracotta
dish (it must not be metal)
and sprinkle with salt.
3. Heat the oil in a heavy-
based pan and gently fry
the garlic and fennel until
soft. Add the vinegar and
wine, bring to the boil and
pour over the sardines,
adding the fennel leaves.
The sardines should be
completely submerged in
the marinade. Cover and
leave in a cold place for at
least 48 hours.
4. Arrange the sardines on
a large platter to serve.

APRIL
An Easter Sunday Buffet Lunch

Serve duck and mango salad and moussaka without meat as alternative main courses. Guests who are watching their calories more sternly should opt for the moussaka, which is a low fat, meatless version of the popular Greek recipe and has far fewer calories than the duck.
Menu serves 8.

Yellow, Red and Green Stuffed Peppers

2 tablespoons olive oil
225 g (8 oz) long-grain rice
8 tablespoons chicken stock
275 g (10 oz) fresh spinach, trimmed
175 g (6 oz) Feta or white Stilton cheese, crumbled
25 g (1 oz) basil or mint, chopped
2 teaspoons dried dill
1 egg, beaten
freshly ground black pepper
8 red, green or yellow peppers
2 tablespoons lemon juice

PREPARATION TIME:
25 minutes
COOKING TIME:
1 hour 25 minutes
OVEN TEMPERATURE:
190°C, 375°F, Gas Mark 5
CALORIES PER PORTION:
260 (1560 kilojoules)

1. Heat 1 tablespoon of the oil over a gentle heat. Add the rice and toss until thoroughly coated. Add the chicken stock. Simmer uncovered until all the liquid has been absorbed. The rice will now be only partially cooked.
2. Finely chop the spinach and mix it with the crumbled Feta cheese, basil, dill and beaten egg. Add pepper to taste and combine with the cooled rice.
3. Wipe the peppers thoroughly with paper towels and cut off the tops to make lids. Use scissors to snip down and inside to loosen all the seeds, but take care not to pierce the sides. Remove the seeds.
4. Fill each pepper with the rice mixture, replace the lids and stand them, tightly packed together, in a casserole with a lid. Trickle over the remaining tablespoon of oil and the lemon juice and add enough water to come two-thirds of the way up the sides of the casserole.
5. Cover and bake in a preheated oven for about 1¼ hours. Serve warm or cold.

Moussaka

1.25 kg (2¾ lb) aubergines
salt
1 tablespoon sunflower oil
2 large onions, peeled and chopped
15 g (½ oz) butter
1 tablespoon cornflour
900 ml (1½ pints) plain unsweetened yogurt
450 g (1 lb) ripe tomatoes, peeled, skinned and chopped
freshly ground black pepper
½ teaspoon ground cinnamon
50 g (2 oz) grated Parmesan
3 eggs

PREPARATION TIME:
45 minutes, plus draining
COOKING TIME:
about 1 hour
OVEN TEMPERATURE:
200°C, 400°F, Gas Mark 6
CALORIES PER PORTION:
150 (630 kilojoules)

1. Slice ⅔ of the aubergines 1 cm (½ inch) thick, sprinkle them with salt and set aside to drain.
2. Prick the rest of the aubergines all over and boil whole in salted water for 10 minutes.
3. Pat sliced aubergines dry, paint each slice scantily with oil and grill until lightly coloured; drain.
4. Soften the onions in the melted butter. Mix the cornflour into the yogurt.
5. Peel the whole aubergines and mash them, mix with the onions, tomatoes, 2 tablespoons of the yogurt mixture, salt, pepper and cinnamon.
6. Line an ovenproof dish with sliced aubergines. Spread some mashed aubergines over and sprinkle with Parmesan. Repeat until the dish is nearly full.
7. Beat the eggs into the remaining yogurt and pour over, sprinkle with a little cinnamon and salt and bake in a preheated oven for 20 minutes.

Duck and Mango Salad

3 duck breast portions, boned
1 bunch spring onions, cut into 2.5 cm (1 inch) lengths
1 celery stick, chopped
1 teaspoon grated orange rind
450 g (1 lb) brown rice, cooked
salt
freshly ground black pepper
3 medium ripe mangoes, peeled and sliced
Sauce:
1 egg yolk
1 whole egg
1 teaspoon Dijon mustard
1 tablespoon mango chutney
½ tablespoon soy sauce
1 tablespoon light vinegar, preferably a fruit vinegar
2 tablespoons corn and sunflower oil mixed
250 ml (8 fl oz) plain unsweetened yogurt

PREPARATION TIME:
25 minutes, plus cooling
COOKING TIME:
20 minutes
OVEN TEMPERATURE:
230°C, 450°F, Gas Mark 8
CALORIES PER PORTION:
375 (1575 kilojoules)

1. Arrange the duck breasts, skin side up, on a rack and roast in a preheated oven for 10 minutes on each side.
2. When cold, remove the skin and cube the meat.
3. In the meantime, make the sauce. Place the egg yolk, whole egg, mustard, chutney, soy sauce and vinegar in a food processor and combine. Add the oil in a very slow trickle, then add the yogurt, a tablespoon at a time.
4. In a large bowl combine the duck meat with the onions, celery, orange rind, cooked rice and seasoning.
5. Arrange the mango slices on top of the salad and serve, accompanied by the sauce.

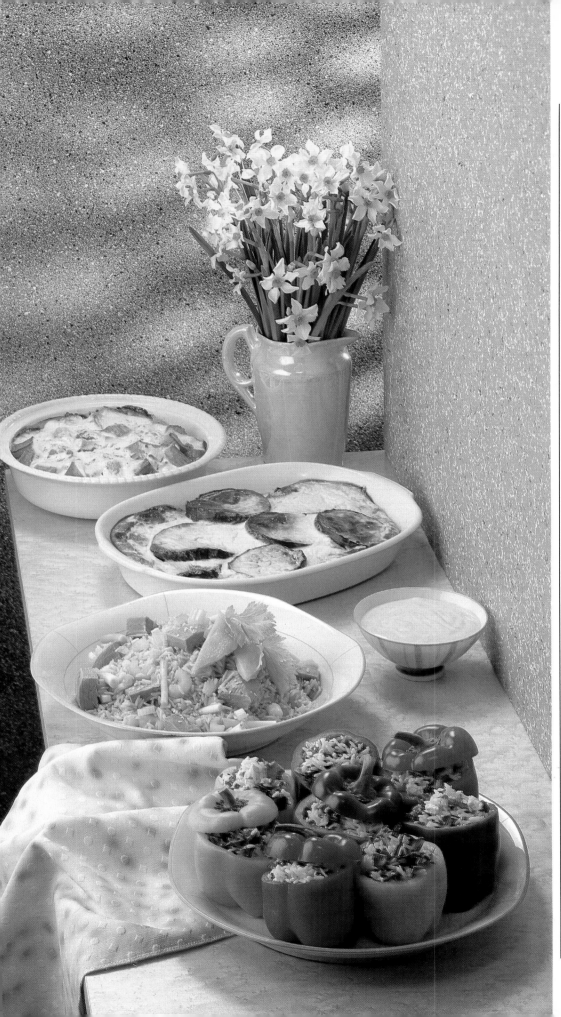

Rhubarb and Hazelnut Dessert

450 g (1 lb) fresh young
  rhubarb
1 tablespoon honey
100 g (4 oz) shelled whole
  hazelnuts
2 eggs (size 1)
1 teaspoon caster sugar
600 ml (1 pint) plain
  unsweetened yogurt
½ teaspoon ground cinnamon

PREPARATION TIME:
10 minutes
COOKING TIME:
50 minutes
OVEN TEMPERATURE:
160°C, 325°F, Gas Mark 3
CALORIES PER PORTION:
130 (550 kilojoules)

The dish works best when served cold but not chilled.

1. Wash and trim the rhubarb, slice it into 5 mm (¼ inch) lengths, place it in a bowl and mix in the honey.
2. Dry-fry or toast the hazelnuts until dark brown, but not burnt. Lightly grind them (or chop them very finely) and combine with the rhubarb.
3. Whisk the eggs, adding the sugar, and combine with the yogurt.
4. Put the fruit and nut mixture in a shallow ovenproof dish, press it down as much as possible and smooth the surface; pour over the yogurt mixture and sprinkle the top with the cinnamon.
5. Bake in a preheated oven for about 45 minutes. Serve cold.

FROM THE TOP Rhubarb and hazelnut dessert; Moussaka; Duck and mango salad; Yellow, red and green stuffed peppers

APRIL

Hors d'oeuvres and Light Meals

Pasta and Bean Salad

2 tablespoons olive oil
3 tablespoons unsweetened orange juice
1 garlic clove, peeled and crushed
salt
freshly ground black pepper
2 tablespoons finely chopped fresh parsley
175 g (6 oz) wholewheat pasta shapes
175 g (6 oz) cooked red kidney beans
50 g (2 oz) soya bean sprouts
2 tablespoons plain unsweetened yogurt
1 tablespoon chopped chives
75 g (3 oz) alfalfa salad sprouts

PREPARATION TIME:
15 minutes, plus cooling
COOKING TIME:
8–10 minutes
CALORIES PER PORTION:
260 (1090 kilojoules)

Both soya bean sprouts and alfalfa salad sprouts can be found in supermarkets that stock a good selection of vegetables, and in health food stores. Alternatively, they can easily be grown at home. Soak 2 tablespoons of beans in water overnight then drain and put in a clean jam jar. Fill the jar with water and leave in a dark place for 4 days, rinsing the beans and changing the water every day.

1. Mix the olive oil with the orange juice, garlic, salt and pepper to taste and the chopped parsley.
2. Cook the wholewheat pasta shapes in a large pan of boiling salted water until tender (8–10 minutes, depending on the size of the pasta shapes).
3. Drain the pasta shapes thoroughly and stir into the orange and oil dressing while the pasta is still warm. Allow to cool.
4. Mix in the kidney beans and soya bean sprouts; stir in the yogurt and chives.
5. Spoon the prepared salad on to a shallow serving dish and arrange the alfalfa salad sprouts around the edge. Serve as a complete light meal.

Cauliflower Ramekins

1 small cauliflower
salt
3 tablespoons wholemeal breadcrumbs
2 tablespoons plain unsweetened yogurt
1 tablespoon chopped fresh dill
2 eggs, separated
2 tablespoons grated Parmesan cheese
1 teaspoon Pesto sauce
freshly ground black pepper
sprigs of fresh dill, to garnish

PREPARATION TIME:
20–25 minutes
COOKING TIME:
about 25 minutes
OVEN TEMPERATURE:
190°C, 375°F, Gas Mark 5
CALORIES PER PORTION:
100 (420 kilojoules)

1. Trim off the leaves and base stalk from the cauliflower (reserve and use for soup). Divide the cauliflower into florets and cook in boiling salted water until just tender. Drain and mash to a purée.
2. Put the purée into a pan and stir over a gentle heat for 1–2 minutes; this will allow some of the excess moisture to evaporate.
3. Mix the purée with the breadcrumbs, yogurt, dill, egg yolks, half the Parmesan cheese, Pesto sauce and salt and pepper to taste.
4. Whisk the egg whites until stiff but not dry; fold lightly but thoroughly into the cauliflower mixture.
5. Spoon into 4 greased ramekin dishes then sprinkle with the remaining Parmesan.
6. Bake in the oven for about 15–20 minutes, until puffed and lightly golden.
7. Serve piping hot, garnished with fresh dill.

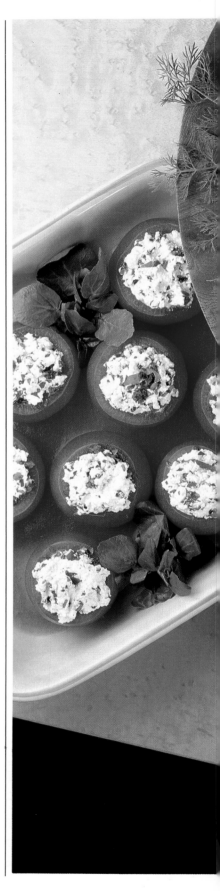

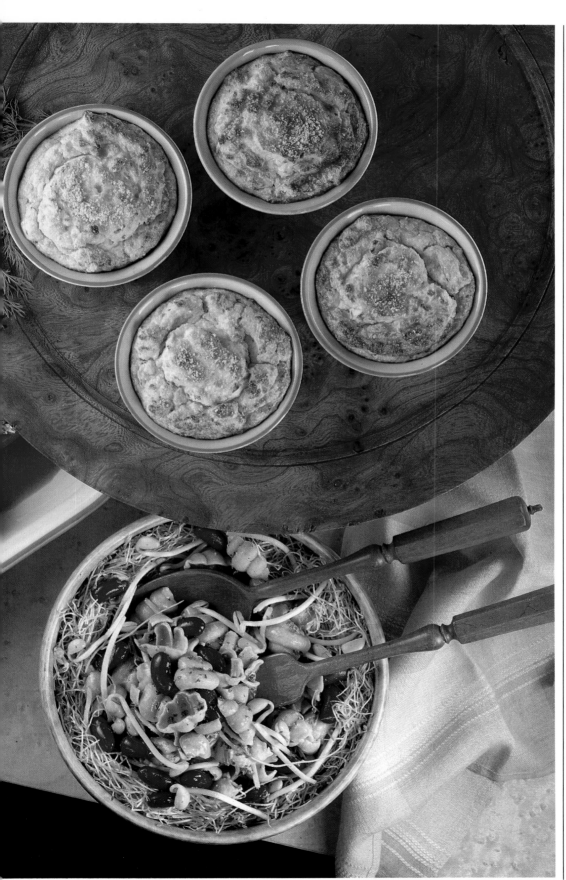

Watercress-stuffed Tomatoes

8 firm tomatoes
275 g (10 oz) cottage cheese,
  sieved
1 garlic clove, peeled and
  crushed
salt
freshly ground black pepper
1 bunch watercress, washed,
  dried and very finely
  chopped
2 tablespoons tomato juice
1 tablespoon dry sherry
small sprigs of watercress, to
  garnish

PREPARATION TIME:
30–35 minutes
CALORIES PER PORTION:
90 (380 kilojoules)

1. Cut a thin slice from the stalk end of each tomato; using a teaspoon, scoop out the centre pulp from each tomato into a bowl, hollowing out as much as possible without breaking the skin.
2. Fill the tomato shells with crumpled paper towels to absorb excess moisture.
3. Mix the cottage cheese with the garlic, salt and pepper to taste, and the chopped watercress; remove the paper towels and fill each hollowed tomato with this mixture.
4. Push the tomato pulp through a sieve, and mix with the tomato juice and sherry.
5. Arrange the stuffed tomatoes on a serving dish; spoon the tomato and sherry sauce around them and garnish with sprigs of watercress.

CLOCKWISE FROM BOTTOM Pasta and bean salad; Watercress-stuffed tomatoes; Cauliflower ramekins

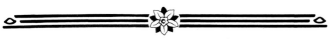

APRIL

Main Courses

Broccoli Soufflé

450 g (1 lb) broccoli
salt
2 tablespoons butter
2 tablespoons plain flour
150 ml (¼ pint) skimmed
 milk
3 tablespoons dry white wine
freshly ground black pepper
4 eggs, separated
3 anchovy fillets, chopped
3 tablespoons grated
 Parmesan cheese
2 tablespoons wholemeal
 breadcrumbs

PREPARATION TIME:
15–20 minutes
COOKING TIME:
45–50 minutes
OVEN TEMPERATURE:
190°C, 375°F, Gas Mark 5
CALORIES PER PORTION:
355 (1490 kilojoules)

1. Cook the broccoli in
boiling salted water until
quite tender. Drain very
thoroughly and liquidize.
2. Heat the butter in a pan;
stir in the flour and cook
for 1 minute. Gradually stir
in the milk and wine; bring
to the boil, stirring until
the sauce has thickened.
3. Stir in the broccoli
purée, salt and pepper to
taste, egg yolks, anchovy
fillets and 2 tablespoons of
the Parmesan cheese.
4. Grease a 1.5 litre (2½
pint) soufflé dish and
sprinkle with breadcrumbs.
5. Whisk the egg whites
until stiff but not dry; fold
lightly but thoroughly into
the broccoli mixture.
Transfer to the prepared
soufflé dish and sprinkle
with the remaining cheese.
6. Bake in the oven for 25–
30 minutes, until risen and
golden. The soufflé will not
rise as high as a standard
soufflé. Serve immediately.

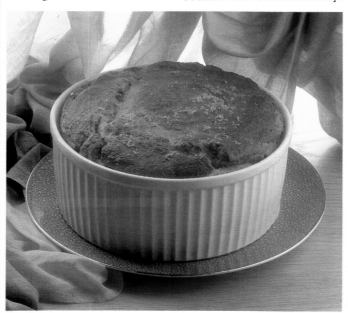

Piquant Plaice

8 small plaice fillets, skinned,
 about 65 g (2½ oz) each
salt
freshly ground black pepper
¼ teaspoon ground ginger
1 small onion, peeled and
 finely chopped
150 ml (¼ pint) white wine
150 ml (¼ pint) chicken stock
2 green leeks, cleaned and cut
 into matchstick strips
4 tablespoons low calorie
 mayonnaise
4 tablespoons plain
 unsweetened yogurt
1 thin slice fresh ginger
½ teaspoon mild curry
 powder
small croûtons, to garnish

PREPARATION TIME:
20 minutes
COOKING TIME:
13 minutes
CALORIES PER PORTION:
200 (835 kilojoules)

1. Lay the plaice fillets
down, skinned sides
uppermost, and sprinkle
with salt, pepper and
ginger. Roll up and secure
with wooden cocktail
sticks.
2. Scatter the onion in a
large frying pan; lay the
plaice on the top and add
the white wine and stock.
Cover the pan and simmer
gently for about 10
minutes.
3. Meanwhile simmer the
strips of leek in boiling
water for 3 minutes.
4. Remove the plaice
paupiettes and keep warm.
Place the drained strips of
leek around the fish.
5. Mix the mayonnaise
with the yogurt. Squeeze
the ginger in a garlic press to
extract the juice and add to
the mixture with the curry
powder and seasonings.
6. Arrange 2 paupiettes on
each plate and garnish
with the strips of leek and
croûtons. Serve the sauce
separately.

Pork Medallions with Parsley Purée

15 g (½ oz) butter
1 small onion, peeled and
 finely chopped
1 garlic clove, peeled and
 crushed
100 g (4 oz) coarsely chopped
 fresh parsley
3 tablespoons chicken stock
4 pork medallions, cut from
 the boned and trimmed loin
pinch of ground coriander
salt
freshly ground black pepper

PREPARATION TIME:
10 minutes
COOKING TIME:
about 30 minutes
CALORIES PER PORTION:
250 (1500 kilojoules)

1. Melt the butter in a pan.
Add the onion and garlic
and fry gently for 3
minutes. Add the parsley
and stir over the heat for
1 minute. Add the chicken
stock and simmer for 4
minutes.
2. Put the parsley mixture
into the liquidizer and
blend until smooth.
3. Sprinkle the medallions
of pork with the coriander
and salt and pepper to
taste. Grill until sealed on
one side, then turn the
medallions over and cook
on the other side.
Continue cooking gently
until the pork is tender and
cooked right through.
4. Meanwhile heat the
parsley purée, either in a
covered dish in a
moderately hot oven, or in
a bowl over a pan of
simmering water.
5. Spoon the parsley purée
on to warmed plates and
arrange the cooked
medallions of pork on top.

LEFT Broccoli soufflé RIGHT, FROM
TOP Pork medallions with parsley
purée; Piquant plaice

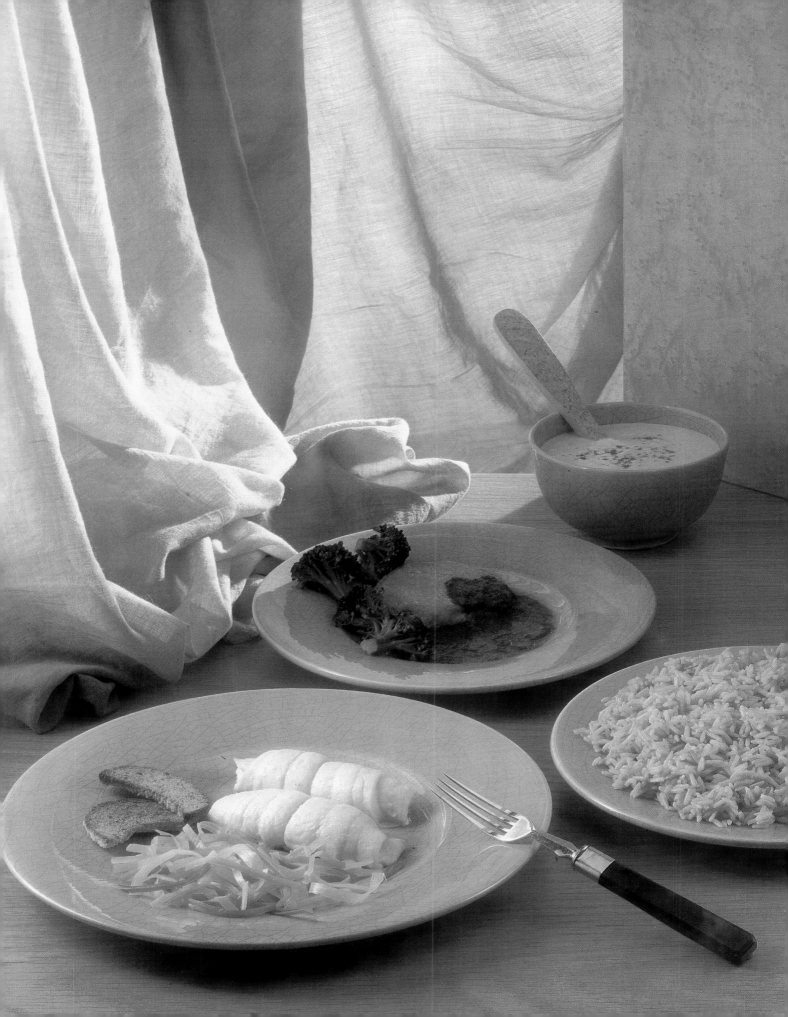

APRIL

Puddings

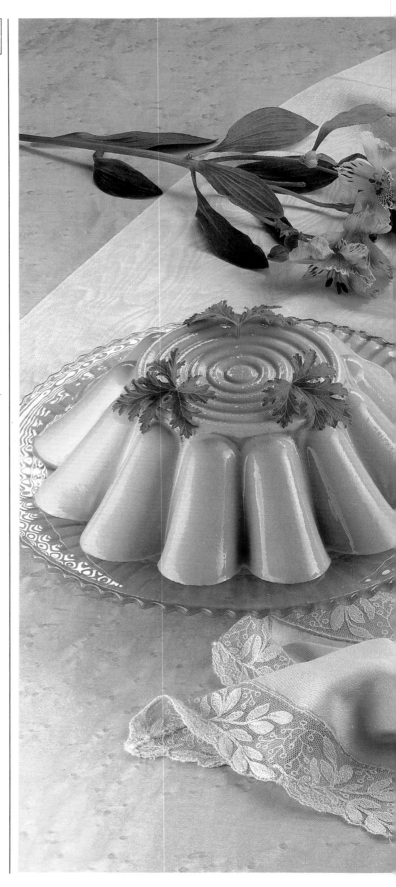

Curd Cheese Hearts

225 g (8 oz) cottage cheese, sieved
artificial sweetener, to taste
150 ml (¼ pint) plain unsweetened yogurt
2 egg whites
1 tablespoon brandy
To decorate:
tiny fresh vine leaves (if available)
small clusters of black grapes

PREPARATION TIME:
30 minutes, plus chilling
CALORIES PER PORTION:
220 (915 kilojoules)

1. Mix the cottage cheese with a little sweetener to taste (if you don't have a very sweet tooth, this may not be necessary); blend in the yogurt.
2. Whisk the egg whites until stiff but not dry; fold lightly but thoroughly into the cheese mixture together with the brandy.
3. Line 4 small perforated heart-shaped moulds with clean muslin; spoon the cheese mixture into the lined moulds and cover with another layer of muslin.
4. Place the moulds on a tray or baking sheet with a rim, and chill for 6–8 hours; the excess liquid should have drained away from the cheese, and the moulds should be firm enough to turn out.
5. Unmould the hearts and decorate with vine leaves and clusters of grapes.

Coffee Yogurt Cream

150 ml (¼ pint) strong black coffee
artificial sweetener, to taste
300 ml (½ pint) plain unsweetened yogurt
150 ml (¼ pint) skimmed milk
3 teaspoons powdered gelatine
3 tablespoons water
lemon-scented geranium leaves, to garnish

PREPARATION TIME:
15 minutes, plus chilling
CALORIES PER PORTION:
65 (270 kilojoules)

This is delicious with wedges of peeled ripe pear.

1. Mix the black coffee with sweetener to taste; add the yogurt and milk.
2. Dissolve the gelatine in the 3 tablespoons water and add to the coffee mixture; mix thoroughly.
3. Pour into 1 lightly oiled large fluted mould, or 4 individual ones, and chill for about 2 hours until set.
4. Carefully unmould the cream on to a flat serving plate; decorate with lemon-scented geranium leaves and serve.

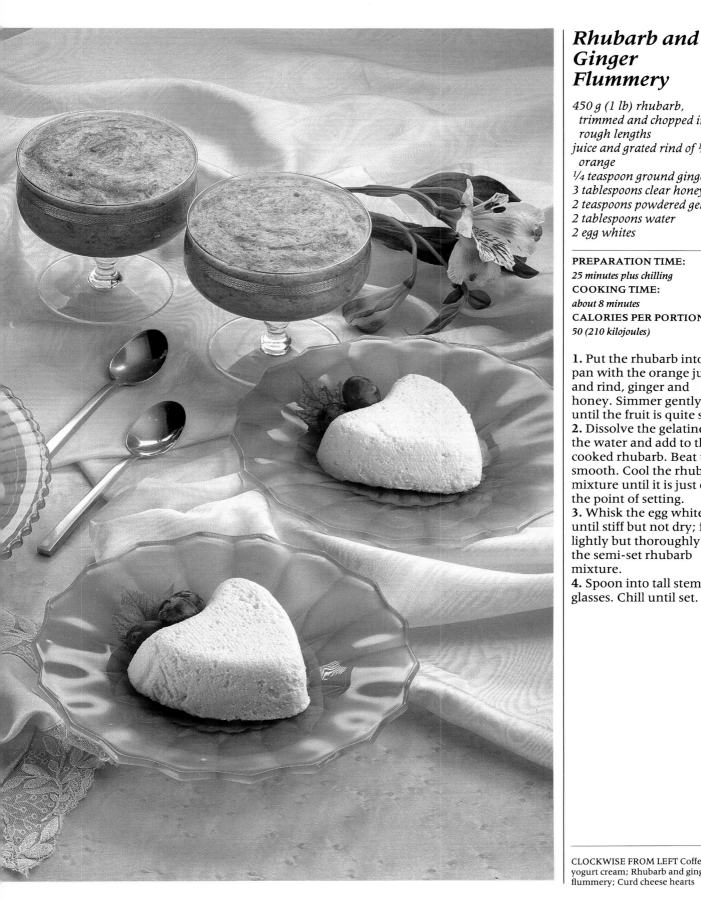

Rhubarb and Ginger Flummery

450 g (1 lb) rhubarb,
  trimmed and chopped into
  rough lengths
juice and grated rind of ½
  orange
¼ teaspoon ground ginger
3 tablespoons clear honey
2 teaspoons powdered gelatine
2 tablespoons water
2 egg whites

PREPARATION TIME:
25 minutes plus chilling
COOKING TIME:
about 8 minutes
CALORIES PER PORTION:
50 (210 kilojoules)

1. Put the rhubarb into a pan with the orange juice and rind, ginger and honey. Simmer gently until the fruit is quite soft.
2. Dissolve the gelatine in the water and add to the cooked rhubarb. Beat until smooth. Cool the rhubarb mixture until it is just on the point of setting.
3. Whisk the egg whites until stiff but not dry; fold lightly but thoroughly into the semi-set rhubarb mixture.
4. Spoon into tall stemmed glasses. Chill until set.

CLOCKWISE FROM LEFT Coffee yogurt cream; Rhubarb and ginger flummery; Curd cheese hearts

APRIL

Dinner Party for Six

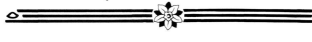

Baba Ghanoush

1 kg (2 lb) aubergines
2–3 tablespoons lemon juice
3 garlic cloves, peeled and
  very finely chopped
1 teaspoon salt
3 tablespoons tahini (sesame
  seed paste)
1 tablespoon finely chopped
  fresh parsley or
½ tablespoon finely chopped
  fresh coriander
sprigs of fresh parsley, to
  garnish

PREPARATION TIME:
10 minutes
COOKING TIME:
30 minutes
OVEN TEMPERATURE:
200°C, 400°F, Gas Mark 6
CALORIES PER PORTION:
110 (460 kilojoules)

1. Prick the aubergines all over and bake for approximately 20 minutes.
2. Heat the grill or a griddle pan and continue to cook the aubergines, turning them until the skins are completely charred. Cool slightly then cut in half and scoop out the flesh.
3. Purée the aubergine with the lemon juice.
4. Mash the garlic with the salt in a pestle and mortar, and add to the purée. Stir in the tahini; leave to cool.
5. When cold, stir in the parsley or coriander.
6. Garnish with parsley sprigs and serve.

Fresh and Smoked Seafood Pie

2 red peppers, seeded and
  roughly chopped
1 tablespoon oil
1 medium fresh mackerel
1 small fillet smoked
  mackerel, about 100 g (4 oz)
1 Finnan haddock
fresh haddock, the same
  weight as the Finnan
1 teaspoon tomato purée
1 tablespoon wine vinegar
40 g (1½ oz) unsalted butter
40 g (1½ oz) plain flour
4 tablespoons skimmed milk
2 large fresh garlic cloves,
  peeled and finely chopped
2 tablespoons finely chopped
  parsley
450 g (1 lb) seasoned mashed
  potatoes
To garnish:
2 unpeeled prawns
5–6 canned baby clams

PREPARATION TIME:
45–55 minutes
COOKING TIME:
about 1 hour
OVEN TEMPERATURE:
200°C, 400°F, Gas Mark 6
CALORIES PER PORTION:
343 (1440 kilojoules)

1. Sweat the chopped peppers in the oil, covered, over a gentle heat until very soft.
2. Meanwhile, bone all the fish then cut up the raw fish. Flake the smoked fish and keep separate.
3. Make fish stock with the fish trimmings by boiling them in 600 ml (1 pint) water until reduced to 300 ml (½ pint).
4. Push the cooked red pepper through a sieve or vegetable mill into a larger pan, add the tomato purée and vinegar, bring to boiling point and add the raw fish. Stir, cover and cook gently for 3 minutes.
5. Melt the butter in a saucepan, stir in the flour and when thoroughly combined stir in the strained fish stock, then the milk. Cook, stirring, to make a smooth sauce.
6. Combine the sauce with the partly cooked fresh fish in a large shallow pie dish. Carefully fold in the flaked smoked fish, garlic and the parsley.
7. Cover with the mashed potato.
8. Bake in a preheated oven for 25 minutes or until it begins to bubble and the top has browned.
9. Garnish with unpeeled prawns and baby clams and serve with a green salad.

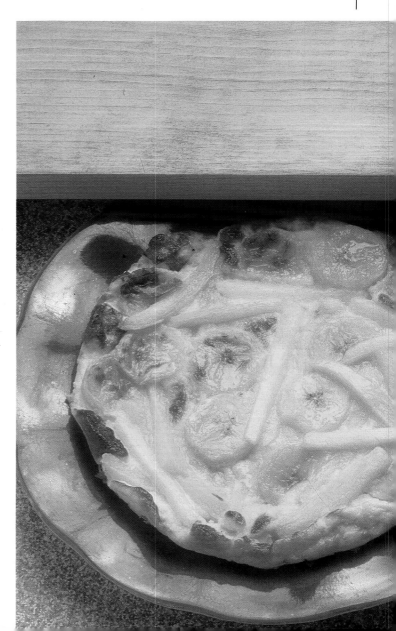

Baked Sweet Omelette

6 eggs
pinch of salt
2 tablespoons plain
  unsweetened yogurt
1 dessert pear
1 tablespoon lemon juice
1 mango
1 banana
1 teaspoon clear honey
1 teaspoon butter

PREPARATION TIME:
15 minutes
COOKING TIME:
about 10 minutes
OVEN TEMPERATURE:
230°C, 450°F, Gas Mark 8
CALORIES PER PORTION:
140 (590 kilojoules)

1. Whisk the eggs with the salt until light and frothy, add the yogurt and whisk again.
2. Peel the pear and cut it into small strips (the same size as French fries), put in a bowl and sprinkle with the lemon juice.
3. Peel and cut the mango in the same way, peel and slice the banana. Combine in a bowl and stir in the honey.
4. Melt the butter in a flameproof and ovenproof dish or a frying pan with heatproof handle. Pour in the egg mixture and stir for 1 minute, then add the fruit, distributing it evenly by stirring gently.
5. When the bottom of the omelette is just beginning to set, transfer it to a preheated oven and bake for approximately 8 minutes or until set to your liking.
6. Serve at once, cut into wedges.

FROM THE LEFT Baked sweet omelette; Baba ghanoush; Fresh and smoked seafood pie

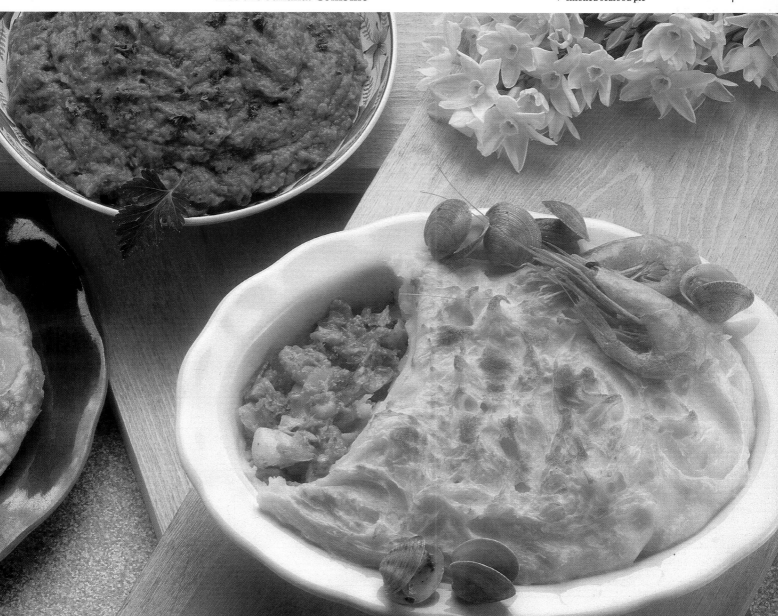

MAY
Bank Holiday Brunch for Six

Brunch is a marvellous meal, almost anything goes, and what a time to entertain, too! You may not wish to serve both the gnocchi and the kedgeree, unless you are going to entertain more than 6 people.

Citrus Fruit Salad

2 limes, peeled and thinly sliced
1 small lemon, peeled and segmented
4 sweet oranges, peeled and coarsely chopped
4 mandarins, peeled and coarsely chopped
2–3 grapefruit, peeled and coarsely chopped
1 teaspoon granulated sugar
1 teaspoon Angostura bitters
3 tablespoons sparkling mineral water
12 kumquats (optional)
1 bunch fresh mint
shredded mint leaves, to garnish

PREPARATION TIME:
45–55 minutes, plus chilling
CALORIES PER PORTION:
80 (335 kilojoules)

If the salad is too sharp, add 1 tablespoon honey, heated slightly so that it mixes easily. This will increase the calorie count to 95 (400 kilojoules) per portion.

1. Using a potato peeler, take a wafer-thin sliver from the discarded skins of all the citrus fruit except the kumquats.
2. Using a pestle and mortar, crush the slivers with the sugar to release the highly flavoured oils, combine with the Angostura bitters and mineral water and set aside.
3. Place the fruit in a deep bowl. Halve the unpeeled kumquats and add them. Strain the mineral water and stir it in.
4. Plunge the bunch of fresh mint, tied with a piece of thread, in and out of boiling water, then straight into the fruit. Chill, covered, for 2 hours.
5. Remove the mint before serving and stir in the shredded mint leaves.

Potato Gnocchi

750 g (1½ lb) large floury potatoes, washed
200 g (7 oz) plain flour
1 egg, lightly beaten
salt
1 teaspoon melted butter
300 ml (½ pint) plain unsweetened yogurt
To serve, either:
1 tablespoon sesame seeds, dry-fried
1 tablespoon clear honey
or
75 g (3 oz) mature Cheddar, finely grated
4 tomatoes, sliced and grilled

PREPARATION TIME:
20–40 minutes
COOKING TIME:
30 minutes
OVEN TEMPERATURE:
200°C, 400°F, Gas Mark 6
CALORIES PER PORTION:
300 (1270 kilojoules), for sesame/honey variation
365 (1525 kilojoules), for Cheddar/tomato variation

1. Prick the potatoes in several places and bake them in their skins for about 1 hour.
2. Cool slightly, scoop all the potato out of the skins and, while still hot, push it through a sieve or the finest disc of a vegetable mill on to a floured surface.
3. When cooled, make a well in the middle, and add the flour, egg and salt, to taste. With your fingers work the flour and egg together with the potato; you may need a little extra flour, depending on the moisture content of the potatoes.
4. When all the ingredients are well blended, lightly knead the mixture until you have a smooth dough. Keep your hands well floured.
5. Divide the dough into manageable portions and form sausage shapes about

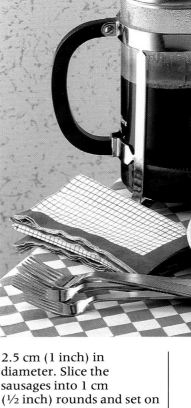

2.5 cm (1 inch) in diameter. Slice the sausages into 1 cm (½ inch) rounds and set on a floured surface, not touching each other.
6. Bring a large saucepan of water to the boil and drop in only a few gnocchi at a time. They are cooked when they rise to the surface.
7. Carefully lift them out with a perforated spoon and put them in a warmed lightly buttered serving dish. When they are all cooked, drizzle the melted butter over.
8. To serve, either melt the honey and drizzle over the gnocchi, then scatter the sesame seeds on top, or sprinkle the gnocchi with grated cheese and accompany with grilled tomato slices. In both cases, serve with a bowl of plain unsweetened yogurt.

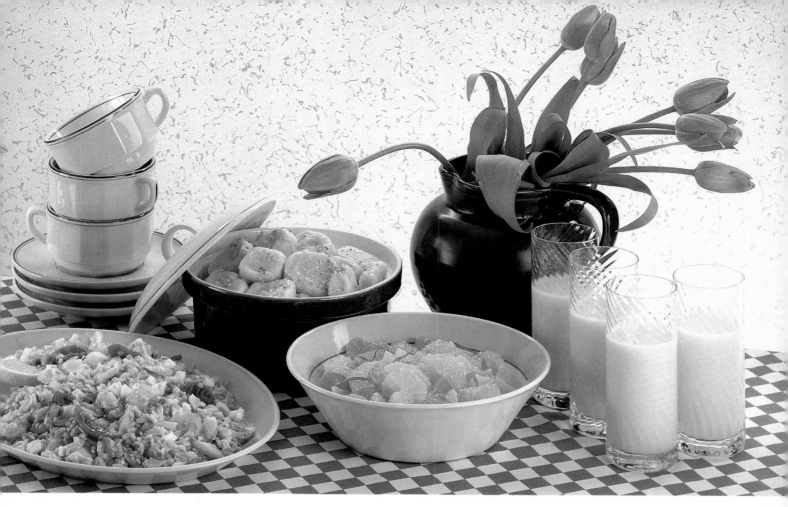

Lentil and Brown Rice Kedgeree

100 g (4 oz) brown rice
salt
100 g (4 oz) orange lentils
1 tablespoon corn, sunflower, soya or olive oil
1 garlic clove, peeled and finely sliced
1 teaspoon cumin seed
1 teaspoon black mustard seed
3 hard-boiled eggs, shelled
1 tablespoon lime pickle
750 g (1½ lb) cooked smoked haddock, flaked and kept hot
1 tablespoon lemon juice

PREPARATION TIME:
15–20 minutes
COOKING TIME:
30–40 minutes
CALORIES PER PORTION:
300 (1270 kilojoules)

1. Cook the rice in boiling salted water for 30–40 minutes.
2. Put the lentils in a large saucepan of cold unsalted water and bring to the boil, then simmer gently for about 10–15 minutes and taste. They should have a bite to them but not be hard. Strain.
3. When the rice is cooked, drain it and return it to the pan. Fold a teatowel in four, place it over the saucepan, cover it with the lid and keep warm.
4. Heat the oil in a small frying pan and fry the garlic until golden, then add the cumin and black mustard seed and continue frying until the garlic is lightly burnt. Tip the spiced oil over the lentils and mix well.
5. Push the hard-boiled eggs through the coarse disc of a vegetable mill; chop the lime pickle if there are any big pieces in it, combine these with the rice, lentils and flaked haddock in a large warmed serving dish. Sprinkle the lemon juice over and serve warm.

Pineapple Yogurt Drink

900 ml (1½ pints) plain unsweetened yogurt
1 large ripe pineapple, peeled and chopped
300 ml (½ pint) sparkling mineral water
artificial sweetener, to taste

PREPARATION TIME:
10–15 minutes
CALORIES PER PORTION:
150 (620 kilojoules)

A liquidizer or food processor is helpful for this recipe. If you do not have either it will be necessary to poach the pineapple first and push it through a sieve, then whisk it into the yogurt.

1. Place the yogurt and pineapple in a liquidizer or food processor and blend, adding the mineral water. You may need to do this in small quantities at a time, depending on the capacity of your machine.
2. Strain through a very fine sieve into a jug, taste and add artificial sweetener if necessary. Chill thoroughly.

FROM THE LEFT Lentil and brown rice kedgeree; Potato gnocchi; Citrus fruit salad; Pineapple yogurt drink

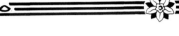

MAY

Hors d'oeuvres and Light Meals

Artichoke Hearts with Orange Vinaigrette

4 globe artichokes
4 tablespoons lemon juice
5 tablespoons orange juice
1 tablespoon olive oil
1 garlic clove, peeled and
  crushed
salt
freshly ground black pepper
4 teaspoons orange lumpfish
  roe
To garnish:
lettuce leaves
sprigs of fresh chervil

PREPARATION TIME:
50 minutes, plus chilling
COOKING TIME:
about 35 minutes
CALORIES PER PORTION:
80 (340 kilojoules)

1. Trim off the stalk close to the base of each artichoke.
2. Bring a large pan of water to the boil and add half the lemon juice; add the prepared artichokes, bring back to the boil and simmer, covered, for 30 minutes until cooked.
3. Meanwhile, make the dressing. Mix the remaining lemon juice with the orange juice, olive oil, garlic and salt and pepper to taste.
4. Remove the artichokes and leave upside down on paper towels to drain.
5. Pull away all the coarse outer leaves from the artichokes, starting from the outside. Once all but the smallest leaves have been removed, you will be able to see the 'choke'.
6. Using a small sharp knife, carefully cut away the choke to expose the artichoke heart; ease the artichoke heart away from the base. Trim the tops of the leaves that are left.
7. Cut the prepared artichoke hearts in half, combine with half of the orange dressing and chill for 30 minutes.
8. Discard the very tiny leaves; scrape the base of each larger leaf to remove the small amount of artichoke flesh. Mix the flesh from the leaves with the remaining dressing. Chill for about 20 minutes.
9. Spoon the artichoke dressing on to 4 small plates; set 2 artichoke halves on each one. Put a spoonful of lumpfish roe into the centre of each.
10. Garnish with lettuce and chervil and serve, accompanied by fingers of brown bread, lightly spread with low fat spread.

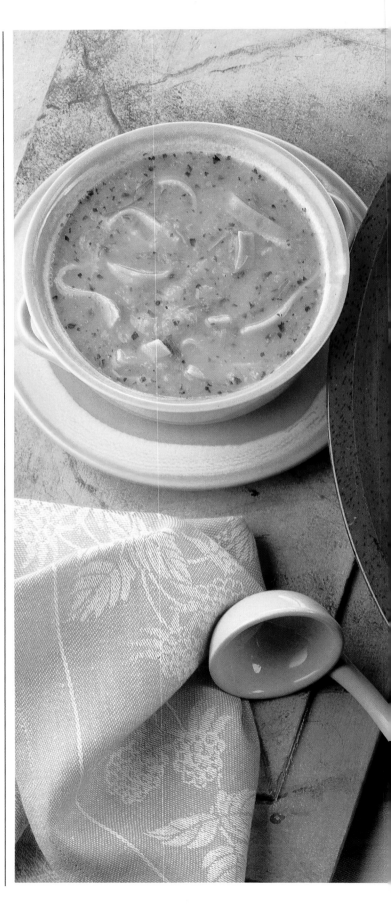

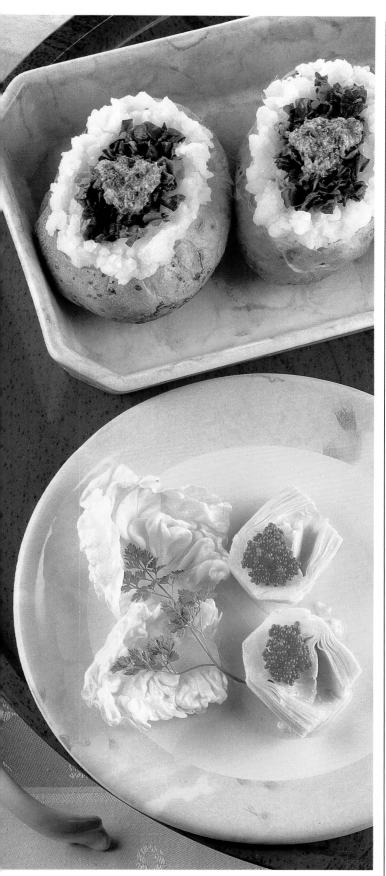

Green Garden Soup

4 celery sticks, chopped
2 leeks, cleaned and chopped
1 bunch watercress, washed
 and chopped
1 heart of a round lettuce,
 shredded
4 spring onions, chopped
1 tablespoon chopped fresh
 tarragon
1 garlic clove, peeled and
 crushed
1 small head fennel, shredded
600 ml (1 pint) chicken stock
300 ml (½ pint) skimmed
 milk
salt
freshly ground black pepper
50 g (2 oz) fine green
 fettucine, broken into short
 lengths

PREPARATION TIME:
15 minutes
COOKING TIME:
about 30 minutes
CALORIES PER PORTION:
90 (375 kilojoules)

1. Put the celery, leeks,
watercress, lettuce, spring
onions, tarragon, garlic,
and fennel into a large
pan; add the stock,
skimmed milk and salt and
pepper to taste.
2. Simmer the soup for
20–25 minutes until all the
vegetables are tender.
3. Blend the soup in the
liquidizer until smooth.
4. Return the soup to a
clean pan and bring to the
boil; add the broken
fettucine and simmer for
about 4 minutes, until the
pasta is just tender. Serve
the soup piping hot.

CLOCKWISE FROM LEFT Green
garden soup; Jacket potatoes with
Pesto; Artichoke hearts with orange
vinaigrette

Jacket Potatoes with Pesto

4 medium baking potatoes,
 about 200 g (7 oz) each
40 g (1½ oz) butter
2 teaspoons Pesto sauce
salt
freshly ground black pepper
generous pinch of ground
 nutmeg
4 tablespoons chopped cooked
 spinach

PREPARATION TIME:
15–20 minutes
COOKING TIME:
1½ hours
OVEN TEMPERATURE:
190°C, 375°F, Gas Mark 5
CALORIES PER PORTION:
320 (1350 kilojoules)

1. Scrub the potatoes and
dry them with paper
towels. Prick each one
several times with a fine
skewer. Wrap each potato
in foil, put into a preheated
oven and bake for 1 hour
20 minutes.
2. Melt the butter; stir in
the Pesto sauce and salt,
pepper and nutmeg to
taste.
3. Remove the potatoes
from the oven and cut a
thin horizontal slice from
the top of each one. Fluff
up the centre potato and
make a slight well in the
centre.
4. Spoon in a little of the
Pesto butter, and then a
spoonful of spinach. Top
with the remaining Pesto
flavoured butter. Pull up
the foil over each filled
potato and return to the
oven for a further 10
minutes.
5. Serve piping hot as a
complete light meal.

MAY

Main Courses

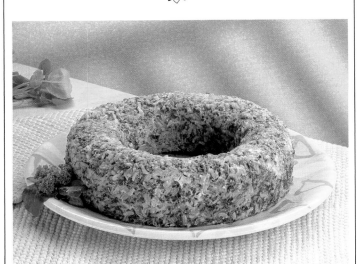

Spring Green and Rice Mould

750 g (1½ lb) spring greens
3 eggs
4 tablespoons plain
  unsweetened yogurt
6 tablespoons cooked brown
  rice
50 g (2 oz) grated Parmesan
  cheese
pinch of ground nutmeg
salt
freshly ground black pepper
1 tablespoon chopped chives
To garnish:
watercress sprigs
parsley sprigs

PREPARATION TIME:
20 minutes
COOKING TIME:
about 50 minutes
OVEN TEMPERATURE:
180°C, 350°F, Gas Mark 4
CALORIES PER PORTION:
185 (775 kilojoules)

1. Wash the greens and shake dry; discard any tough stalk pieces. Shred the greens coarsely and put them into a pan with just enough boiling water to cover the base of the pan; cover and cook gently until they are just tender.
2. Drain the greens thoroughly, pressing to extract as much excess moisture as possible; blend to a purée.
3. Mix the purée with the remaining ingredients. Transfer to a greased 900 ml (1½ pint) mould.
4. Stand the mould in a roasting tin and add sufficient hot water to come half-way up the sides; cover the top of the mould with a circle of lightly greased foil.
5. Bake in a preheated oven for 45 minutes, until the mould is set.
6. Allow to stand for 2–3 minutes, and then carefully turn out on to a plate. Garnish with watercress and parsley.

Baked Salmon with Fennel

4 portions filleted salmon,
  about 150 g (5 oz) each
2 tablespoons lemon juice
4 tablespoons dry white wine
salt
freshly ground black pepper
½ teaspoon fennel seed
1 medium fennel bulb (with
  feathery leaves)
25 g (1 oz) butter
Sauce:
1 egg yolk
1 teaspoon white wine vinegar
150 ml (¼ pint) plain
  unsweetened yogurt

PREPARATION TIME:
20 minutes, plus chilling
COOKING TIME:
25 minutes
OVEN TEMPERATURE:
180°C, 350°F, Gas Mark 4
CALORIES PER PORTION:
190 (770 kilojoules)

1. Put the pieces of salmon fillet into a shallow dish. Add the lemon juice, white wine, salt and pepper to taste, and the fennel seed; cover and chill for 2 hours.
2. Remove the leaves from the fennel and reserve; shred the fennel bulb.
3. Scatter the shredded fennel over the base of a lightly greased shallow ovenproof dish. Lay the pieces of salmon fillet carefully on the top; spoon over the marinade and dot with small knobs of butter.
4. Cover the dish with foil and bake for 20 minutes.
5. Meanwhile make the sauce. Beat the egg yolk with the wine vinegar and the yogurt. Put into the top of a double saucepan and stir over a gentle heat until the sauce has thickened.
6. Arrange the fennel and salmon in a serving dish. Serve the sauce separately in a warmed sauceboat, garnished with the reserved fennel leaves.

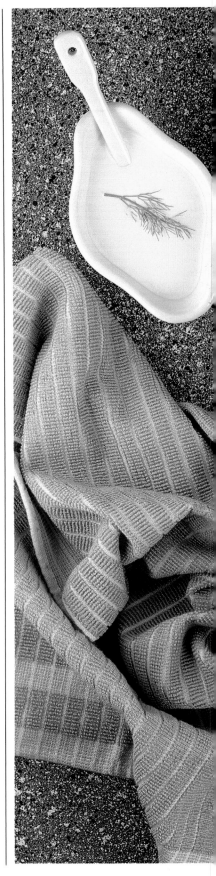

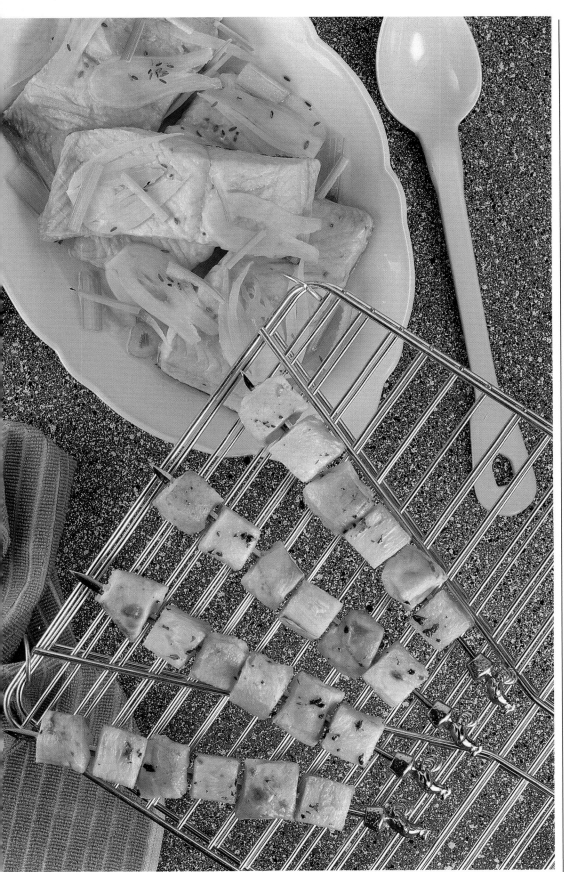

Chicken and Pineapple Kebabs

2 tablespoons olive oil
2 tablespoons unsweetened
  pineapple juice
1 tablespoon lemon juice
1 garlic clove, peeled and
  crushed
salt
freshly ground black pepper
1 tablespoon chopped fresh
  mint
3 boned chicken breasts,
  about 150 g (5 oz) each, cut
  into 2.5 cm (1 inch) cubes
3 large slices fresh pineapple,
  about 225 g (8 oz) total
  weight, peeled and cut into
  2.5 cm (1 inch) cubes

PREPARATION TIME:
20 minutes, plus marinating
COOKING TIME:
10 minutes
CALORIES PER PORTION:
230 (950 kilojoules)

1. Mix the olive oil with
the pineapple juice, lemon
juice, garlic, salt and
pepper to taste and the
chopped mint.
2. Put the cubed chicken
into a shallow dish and
spoon over the prepared
marinade; cover and
marinate for 4 hours.
3. Remove the chicken
from the marinade and
thread on to 4 kebab
skewers alternating with
the pieces of pineapple.
4. Lay the kebabs on the
rack of the grill; brush with
the marinade and cook
under a preheated grill for
4–5 minutes. Turn the
kebabs over, brush once
again with the marinade,
and grill for a further 4–5
minutes, until tender.
5. Serve with cooked
brown rice.

OPPOSITE PAGE Spring green and rice
mould LEFT, FROM TOP Baked
salmon with fennel; Chicken and
pineapple kebabs

MAY

Puddings

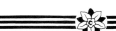

Gooseberry Jelly

450 g (1 lb) gooseberries,
  topped and tailed
150 ml (¼ pint) water
300 ml (½ pint) pure apple
  juice
artificial sweetener, to taste
4 teaspoons powdered gelatine
3 tablespoons dry white wine
fresh angelica leaves or fresh
  gooseberries, to decorate

PREPARATION TIME:
20 minutes, plus chilling
COOKING TIME:
6–8 minutes
CALORIES PER PORTION:
70 (290 kilojoules)

1. Lightly oil a 900 ml (1½ pint) mould.
2. Put the gooseberries into a pan with the water and simmer until soft and pulpy. Blend the fruit in a food processor until smooth.
3. Mix the purée with apple juice and artificial sweetener to taste.
4. Dissolve the gelatine in the white wine and add to the gooseberry mixture; mix thoroughly and pour into the prepared mould. Chill for 2–3 hours until set.
5. Carefully unmould the set jelly on to a serving plate, and decorate with angelica leaves or fresh gooseberries.

Whole Strawberry Ice Cream

3 egg yolks
1 tablespoon redcurrant jelly
1 tablespoon red Vermouth
300 ml (½ pint) plain
  unsweetened yogurt
350 g (12 oz) ripe
  strawberries, hulled
4–6 strawberries with stalks,
  halved, to decorate

PREPARATION TIME:
25 minutes, plus freezing
CALORIES PER PORTION:
155 (650 kilojoules)

1. Put the egg yolks into a food processor with the redcurrant jelly, Vermouth, yogurt, and half the strawberries; blend until smooth.
2. Transfer the mixture to a shallow container, and freeze until the ice cream starts to harden around the edges.
3. Tip the ice cream into a bowl and beat to break up the ice crystals. Chop the remaining strawberries and mix into the semi-set ice cream. Return to the container and freeze until quite firm.
4. Scoop the ice cream into stemmed glasses and decorate each one with strawberry halves.

CLOCKWISE FROM RIGHT
Gooseberry jelly; Whole strawberry ice cream; Apple gâteau

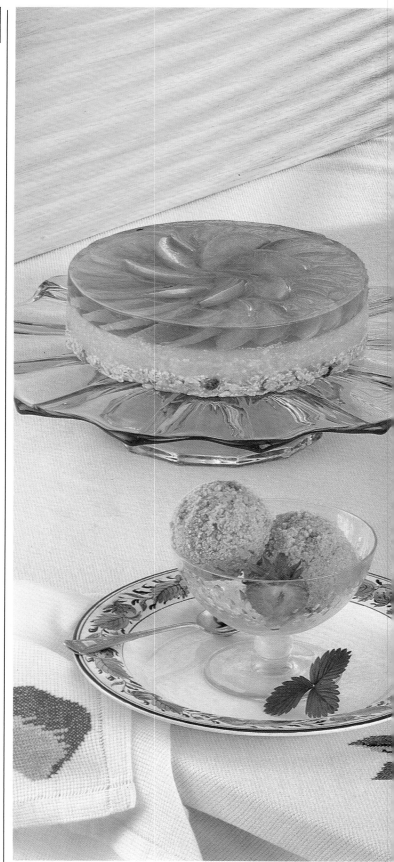

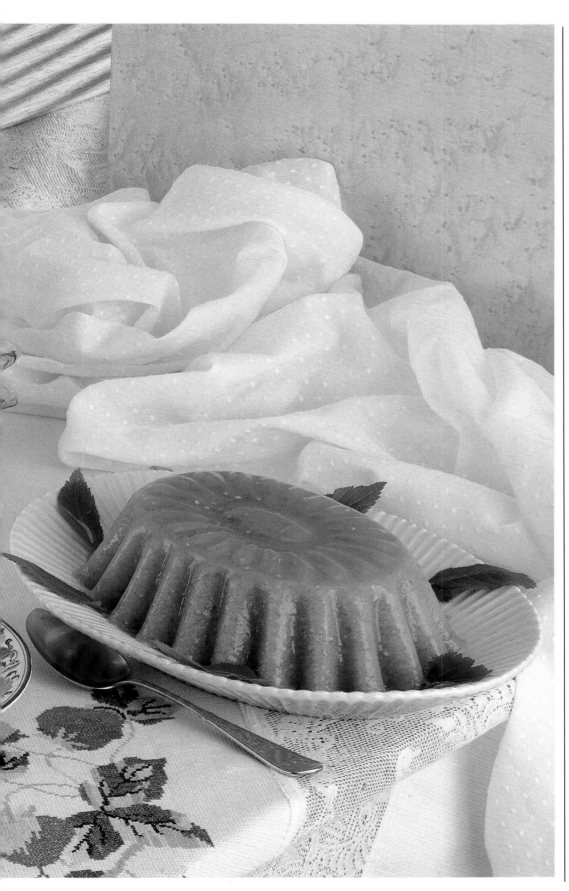

Apple Gâteau

1 sachet powdered gelatine
2 tablespoons water
450 g (1 lb) cooking apples,
  peeled, cored and sliced
juice and grated rind of
  ½ lemon
artificial sweetener, to taste
1 egg yolk
4 tablespoons muesli cereal
25 g (1 oz) low fat spread
2 dessert apples, sliced
150 ml (¼ pint) apple juice

PREPARATION TIME:
30–40 minutes, plus chilling
COOKING TIME:
20 minutes
OVEN TEMPERATURE:
190°C, 375°F, Gas Mark 5
CALORIES PER PORTION:
200 (840 kilojoules)

1. Put half the gelatine and the water in a heatproof bowl and stir over hot water until dissolved.
2. Heat the cooking apples with the lemon rind and juice and a few tablespoons of water until tender. Add sweetener to taste and beat in the yolk. Stir in the dissolved gelatine.
3. Bake the muesli in a preheated oven for 8 minutes. Mix with the low fat spread while still hot.
4. Spread muesli over base of a loose-bottomed 18 cm (7 inch) cake tin. Chill for 30 minutes.
5. Poach the dessert apple slices gently in the apple juice for about 3 minutes; remove carefully and drain on paper towels.
6. Combine the remaining gelatine with 2 tablespoons of apple juice in a heatproof bowl; stir over hot water to dissolve. Stir in remaining apple juice.
7. Spread the apple purée over the muesli base; arrange the apple slices on top. Spoon over the apple juice glaze.
8. Chill for 4 hours.

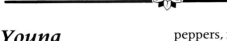

MAY

Dinner Party for Six

Young Vegetables with Garlic Sauce

*about 1.25 kg (2½ lb) raw
and/or cooked vegetables (see
below)*
Sauce:
*3–4 large garlic cloves, peeled
and roughly chopped*
1 teaspoon salt
2–3 tablespoons lemon juice
*4 tablespoons tahini (sesame
seed paste)*
water
*freshly ground black pepper
(optional)*
1 teaspoon olive oil
*2 teaspoons finely chopped
fresh parsley or coriander*

PREPARATION TIME:
about 1½ hours
CALORIES PER PORTION:
150 (620 kilojoules)

Use any of the delicious
seasonal vegetables in the
shops for this dish;
steamed young courgettes,
carrots, baby sweetcorn,
white cabbage and
cauliflower, as well as
salad ingredients such as
peppers, mushrooms and
cucumber. Cold new
potatoes in their skins taste
especially good with the
garlic sauce. Lightly steam
the vegetables or leave
them raw, according to
taste, and choose as
adventurous and colourful
a selection as you can.

1. Prepare the vegetables,
steaming and trimming as
necessary.
2. Using a pestle and
mortar, reduce the garlic to
a pulp with the salt, then
add the lemon juice.
3. Slowly incorporate the
mixture into the tahini,
adding enough water to
make a consistency similar
to thick cream.
4. Taste and adjust the
seasoning with salt, pepper
or lemon juice. Finally stir
in the oil and parsley.
Transfer to a small bowl.
5. Arrange the vegetables
on a platter and place in
the centre of the table. Let
your guests help
themselves to a selection of
vegetables and a spoonful
of garlic sauce.

Veal Pörkölt

*750 g (1½ lb) pie veal in one
piece (boned knuckle of veal
if possible)*
25 g (1 oz) pure lard
*2 large onions, peeled and
finely chopped*
1 tablespoon sweet paprika
½ teaspoon salt
1 tablespoon water
*1 green pepper, halved, cored
and seeded*
1 large tomato, halved
*450 g (1 lb) pasta shells or
noodles, cooked, to serve*

PREPARATION TIME:
8 minutes
COOKING TIME:
about 1 hour
CALORIES PER PORTION:
430 (1810 kilojoules)

1. Cut the meat into large
pieces of about 5 cm
(2 inches).
2. Heat the lard in a heavy-
based saucepan and fry the
onions until golden.
3. Take the pan off the heat
and add the paprika, stir
thoroughly, then add the
meat and return to a gentle
heat. Stir and add the salt
and the water.
4. Cover and simmer
slowly, stirring from time
to time and adding a little
more water should it look
at all dry.
5. After 30 minutes add the
halved green pepper and
tomato, cover and
continue cooking until the
meat is really tender; the
longer and slower the
better.
6. Just before serving,
remove the green pepper,
chop up and combine with
the veal. Turn the pörkölt
into a large warmed
serving dish and surround
with pasta shells. Offer a
simple cucumber salad as
accompaniment.

Grapefruit Glazed in Cointreau

4 large grapefruit, chilled
4 tablespoons orange juice
1 tablespoon honey
½ teaspoon ground nutmeg
2 tablespoons Cointreau
sprig of rosemary, to decorate

PREPARATION TIME:
15 minutes
COOKING TIME:
10 minutes
CALORIES PER PORTION:
55 (230 kilojoules)

1. Peel the grapefruit with
a sharp knife, removing all
the pith at the same time.
Slice into 1 cm (½ inch)
thick rounds.
2. In a large pan heat the
orange juice with the
honey, bring to simmering
point and poach the
grapefruit slices, a few at a
time, for 4–5 minutes. Lift
out with a perforated
spoon and arrange on a
serving dish.
3. When all the grapefruit
slices have been cooked,
add the nutmeg and
Cointreau to the pan, bring
to boiling point and pour it
over the grapefruit.
4. Serve cold, decorated
with a sprig of rosemary.

CLOCKWISE FROM TOP LEFT Veal
pörkölt served with sliced cucumber
salad; Young vegetables with garlic
sauce; Grapefruit glazed in Cointreau

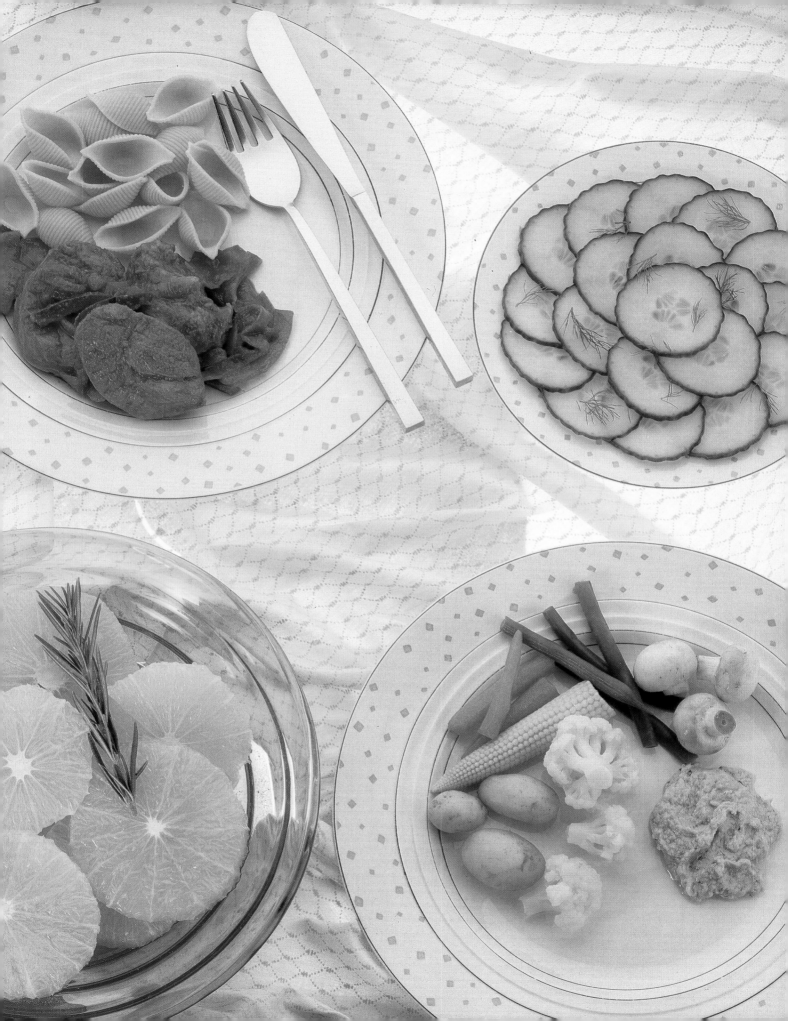

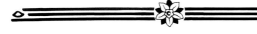

SPRING

Side Salads

Tricolour Salad

100 g (4 oz) leeks, trimmed
and sliced into rings
100 g (4 oz) red pepper, cored,
seeded and diced
2 medium oranges, about
225 g (8 oz) flesh, peeled and
cut into quartered slices
1 tablespoon chopped fresh
dill
1 tablespoon chopped fresh
parsley
150 ml (¼ pint) plain
unsweetened yogurt
1 teaspoon clear honey
freshly ground black pepper

PREPARATION TIME:
10 minutes
CALORIES PER PORTION:
about 55 (215 kilojoules)

Bright colours and
contrasting textures make
this salad a refreshing
antidote to the end of
winter. For the best
flavour, serve at room
temperature, not chilled.

1. Combine the prepared
leeks, red pepper and
oranges in a serving dish.
2. Blend together the dill,
parsley, yogurt, honey and
pepper and pour over the
salad.

Moroccan Salad

25 g (1 oz) blanched split
almonds
1 bunch watercress, coarse
stems removed, washed and
roughly chopped
2 large oranges, about 275 g
(10 oz) flesh, peeled and
thinly sliced
100 g (4 oz) cottage cheese
50 g (2 oz) fresh or dried
dates, roughly chopped
1 teaspoon ground coriander
(optional)

PREPARATION TIME:
10 minutes
CALORIES PER SERVING:
about 115 (485 kilojoules)

A traditional and delicious
combination that makes
the most of the new
season's watercress.

1. Grill the almonds on an
ungreased baking sheet for
2–3 minutes, shaking to
turn them so that they
brown evenly on all sides.
2. Arrange the prepared
watercress and orange
slices around the inside
edge of a serving dish.
3. Either stir in the cottage
cheese, or place it in a neat
mound in the dish.
Arrange the dates and
toasted almonds on top.
4. Sprinkle the salad with
the coriander (if using) and
serve.

Four Fruit Salad

1 orange, peeled and cut into
quartered slices
1 grapefruit, preferably pink,
peeled and segmented and
each segment cut in half
225 g (8 oz) grapes, white or
black, halved and pipped
450 g (1 lb) melon, skin
removed and flesh cut into
balls or small cubes
2 teaspoons finely chopped
fresh mint

PREPARATION TIME:
10 minutes, plus standing
CALORIES PER SERVING:
about 80 (335 kilojoules)

An excellent salad to go
with fish or poultry. By
using white grapes, melon
and grapefruit you can
have subtly similar colours.
Black grapes, yellow-
fleshed melon and pink
grapefruit will give you
vividly contrasting shades.

1. Either arrange the
different fruits in piles on
individual plates and
sprinkle with mint, or
combine all the ingredients
in a serving dish.
2. Allow to stand at room
temperature for 20–30
minutes before serving.

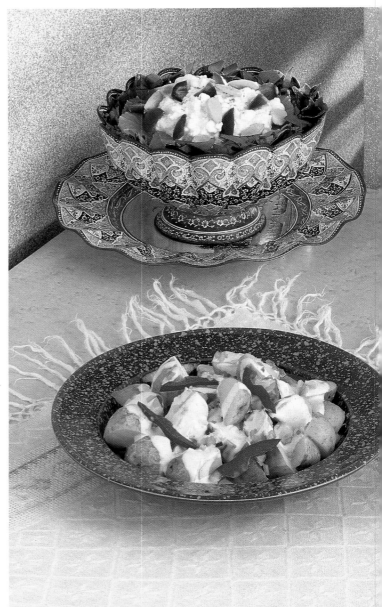

Jacket Potato Salad

350 g (12 oz) small potatoes,
 scrubbed
2–3 spring onions, trimmed
 and finely chopped
150 ml (¼ pint) plain
 unsweetened yogurt
2 tablespoons lemon juice
1 teaspoon mild mustard
pinch of freshly ground black
 pepper
pinch of salt
175 g (6 oz) red peppers,
 cored, seeded and roughly
 sliced

PREPARATION TIME:
5 minutes
COOKING TIME:
30–45 minutes
OVEN TEMPERATURE:
200°C, 400°F, Gas Mark 6
CALORIES PER PORTION:
about 115 (480 kilojoules)

Potatoes can fit into a
slimmer's meal – easily.

1. Thread the potatoes on
to metal kebab skewers.
2. Bake in the preheated
oven for about 30 minutes
or until tender.
3. Stir all the remaining
ingredients except the
peppers together in a
serving dish.
4. Allow the potatoes to
cool slightly, then cut into
rough quarters or cubes
and add to the dish with
the peppers. Toss well and
serve.

CLOCKWISE FROM TOP Moroccan
salad; Four fruit salad; Tricolour salad;
Jacket potato salad

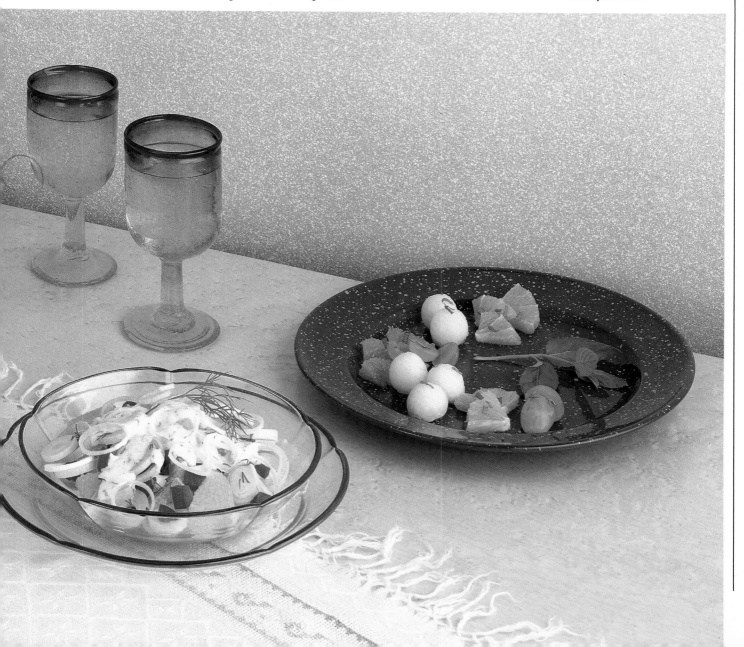

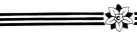

SPRING

Main Course Salads

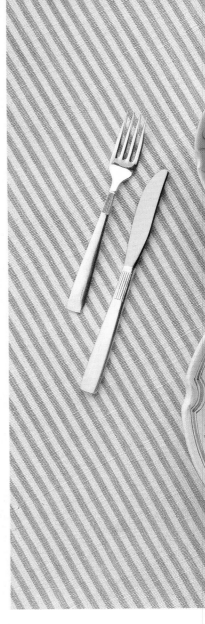

Kipper and Apple Salad

400 g (14 oz) kipper fillets
3 tablespoons lemon juice
2 teaspoons vegetable oil
1 teaspoon ground coriander (optional)
50 g (2 oz) long-grain brown rice, washed
150 ml (¼ pint) water
2 tablespoons chopped fresh parsley
pinch of freshly ground black pepper
175 g (6 oz) red-skinned eating apple
To serve:
1 head of Chinese leaves, about 500 g (1 lb 2 oz)
1 lemon, cut into wedges (optional)

PREPARATION TIME:
10 minutes, plus chilling
COOKING TIME:
about 50 minutes
CALORIES PER SERVING:
about 300 (1255 kilojoules)

A satisfying Scandinavian-style salad to which brown rice supplies fibre.

1. Poach the kipper fillets for 1 minute in simmering water to cover.
2. Drain the kippers, scrape off the skin and cut the fish into bite-size pieces.
3. Place the fish in a glass or pottery dish and pour the lemon juice, oil and coriander (if using) over. Refrigerate for 3–4 hours, stirring occasionally.
4. Bring the rice and water to the boil in a small saucepan. Cover and simmer for 35–45 minutes, until the water has been absorbed and the rice is tender.
5. Combine the rice, preferably while still warm, with the parsley and pepper.
6. To serve, shred the Chinese leaves and divide between 4 dinner plates. Top with spoonfuls of rice. Core and dice the unpeeled apple and arrange on top of the rice on each plate, along with the pieces of kipper. Garnish each plate with a lemon wedge if liked.

Oriental Chicken Salad

750 g (1½ lb) boned chicken
450 ml (¾ pint) water
2 tablespoons wine vinegar
2 teaspoons finely grated orange rind
3 spring onions, trimmed and finely chopped
4 teaspoons soy sauce
1 teaspoon finely grated fresh ginger
2 teaspoons sesame seeds
225 g (8 oz) bean sprouts, rinsed and drained
1 crisp lettuce, washed and torn into shreds

PREPARATION TIME:
10 minutes, plus standing
COOKING TIME:
30–40 minutes
CALORIES PER SERVING:
about 260 (1080 kilojoules)

This unusual oriental dressing will also give a new interest to white fish salads. Crushing the sesame seeds lets out the flavour, which has already been much enhanced by toasting. If you prefer a lot of dressing, double the stock and dressing ingredients.

1. In a medium-size saucepan, bring the chicken and water to the boil. Cover and simmer for 25–30 minutes, until the chicken is cooked through. Turn off the heat and let the chicken cool a little in the stock.
2. Measure out 150 ml (¼ pint) of the stock, and mix with the vinegar, orange rind, spring onions, soy sauce and fresh ginger.
3. Cut the chicken into bite-size pieces, place in a deep serving bowl and pour the dressing over. Leave to stand for at least 30 minutes to allow the flavours to blend.
4. Meanwhile, place the sesame seeds in an ungreased heavy-based pan and stir over a low heat until they start to 'jump' (2–3 minutes). Crush the seeds in an electric coffee mill or with a mortar and pestle.
5. Toss the bean sprouts, lettuce and crushed sesame seeds with chicken, and serve.

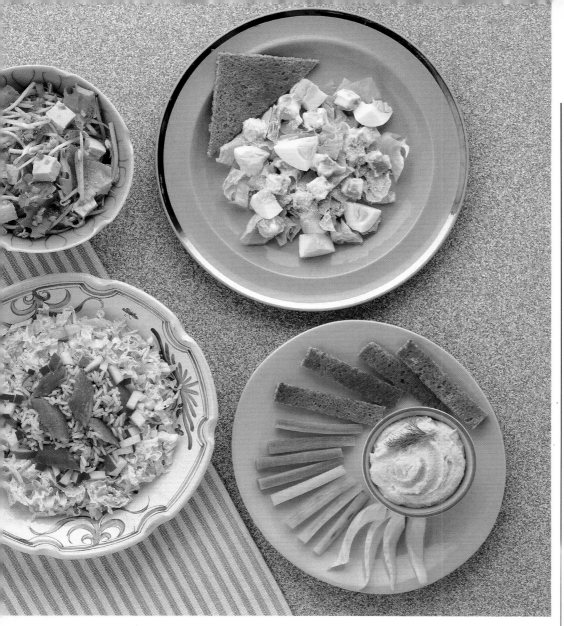

Egg and Bacon Salad

4 eggs (size 1)
100 g (4 oz) lean collar bacon, diced
2 teaspoons wine vinegar
2 teaspoons mild mustard
1 teaspoon clear honey
pinch of salt
250 ml (8 fl oz) plain unsweetened yogurt
1 round lettuce, washed and roughly chopped
2 teaspoons grated Parmesan cheese
4 slices wholemeal bread, about 150 g (5 oz)

PREPARATION TIME:
10 minutes
COOKING TIME:
about 10 minutes
CALORIES PER SERVING:
about 300 (1255 kilojoules)

An unusual warm salad, that will even appeal to those who don't usually like salad.

1. Boil the eggs for 8 minutes.
2. Meanwhile, fry the diced bacon gently in an ungreased heavy-based frying pan until dry. Turn the heat off under the pan and leave the bacon to cool slightly.
3. Add the vinegar, mustard, honey, salt and yogurt to the bacon in the pan. Stir well to mix.
4. Place the lettuce in a serving bowl, pour over the warm bacon dressing and toss.
5. Rinse the eggs under cold water and shell while still warm. Chop them into chunks and stir them into the salad. Sprinkle the Parmesan over.
6. Toast the bread and trim off the crusts. Cut diagonally into triangles. Serve with the salad.

Taramasalata with Crudités

175 g (6 oz) smoked cod's roe
5–6 tablespoons lemon juice
500 g (1 lb 2 oz) low fat soft cheese
¼ teaspoon white pepper
To serve:
175 g (6 oz) carrots, peeled and cut into fingers
175 g (6 oz) wholemeal pitta bread, cut into fingers
275 g (10 oz) cucumber, peeled and cut into fingers
175 g (6 oz) fennel bulb scrubbed and cut into fingers

PREPARATION TIME:
10 minutes, plus chilling (optional)
CALORIES PER SERVING:
about 300 (1255 kilojoules)

Bought taramasalata is very calorific because of its high oil content. This pale pink home-made version is low in fat, and can be reddened with a little beetroot juice if a brighter pink colour is preferred.

1. Scrape the roe from its skin into a mixing bowl.
2. Using a stainless steel fork, mash the roe with half the lemon juice.
3. Blend the cheese into the roe with the pepper. (If using cottage cheese, sieve it finely first.)
4. Taste the mixture and add the remaining lemon juice as necessary.
5. Transfer to 1 large or 4 individual serving bowls.

CLOCKWISE FROM TOP LEFT
Oriental chicken salad; Egg and bacon salad; Taramasalata with crudités; Kipper and apple salad

If possible, chill for about 1 hour.
6. To serve, arrange the vegetable and bread fingers on one large or 4 individual platters and serve with the taramasalata.

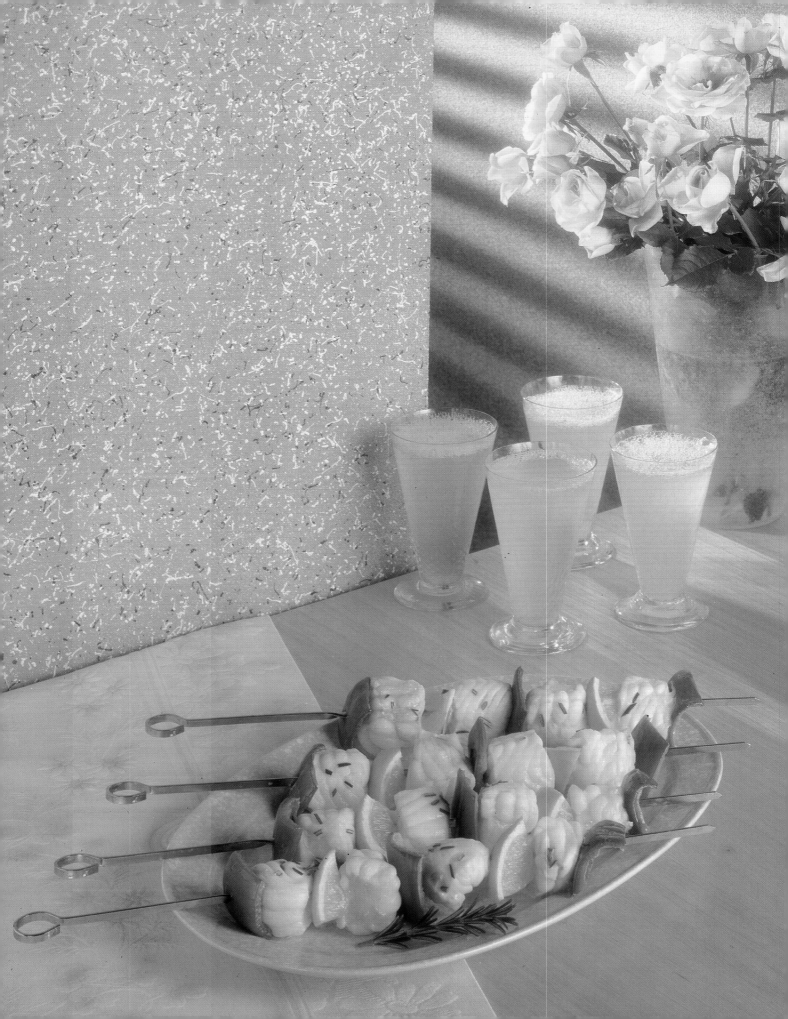

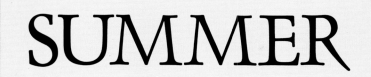

SUMMER

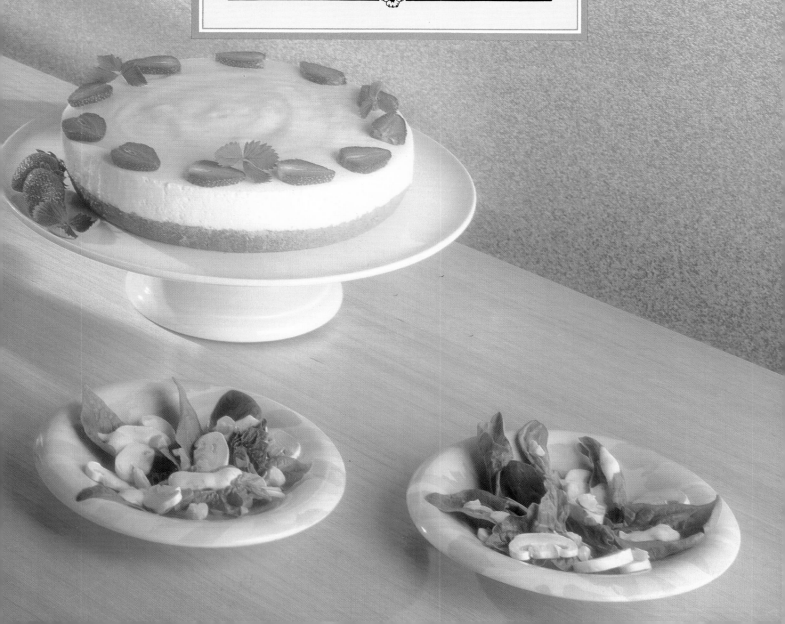

JUNE

Midsummer Party for Ten

Midsummer Day is usually warm enough to allow entertaining out of doors and a cold buffet-style informal meal is ideal for such an occasion.

Zucchini al Forno

5 large or 10 small courgettes, trimmed
salt
1 teaspoon oil
1 garlic clove, peeled and finely chopped
1 × 550 g (20 oz) can tomatoes
1 small can anchovies, drained
1 teaspoon chopped marjoram (fresh or dried)
freshly ground black pepper

PREPARATION TIME:
10–15 minutes, plus cooling
COOKING TIME:
1–1¼ hours
OVEN TEMPERATURE:
200°C, 400°F, Gas Mark 6
CALORIES PER PORTION:
45 (190 kilojoules)

1. Slice the courgettes in half lengthways and scoop out the seeds and seed pulp with a teaspoon. Sprinkle the inside of each courgette with salt and leave to drain upside down on paper towels.
2. Heat the oil in a saucepan and lightly fry the garlic.
3. Push the tomatoes through a vegetable mill or sieve to remove the seeds and add the tomato pulp to the pan. Bring to the boil and cook vigorously until reduced by half. Remove from the heat and stir in one chopped fillet of anchovy and half the marjoram.
4. Wipe the insides of the courgettes with paper towels to remove the salt and set them in a large baking dish; fill each one with tomato sauce and arrange anchovy fillets on top.
5. Grind over plenty of black pepper and bake in a preheated oven for approximately 35–45 minutes. Allow to cool before serving, sprinkled with the remaining marjoram.

Semi-Soused Turkey

1 small turkey, about 3.5 kg (8 lb) (see below)
1 tablespoon green olive oil
2 onions, peeled and finely grated
2 garlic cloves, peeled and grated
bunch of fresh thyme
sprig of fresh sage
sprig of fresh parsley
sprig of fresh marjoram
1 tablespoon salt
1 teaspoon coarsely ground black pepper
½ teaspoon ground allspice
2 tablespoons lemon juice
2 tablespoons wine vinegar
300 ml (½ pint) white wine
1 tablespoon clear honey

PREPARATION TIME:
15 minutes, plus sousing
COOKING TIME:
about 1¾ hours
OVEN TEMPERATURE:
240°C, 475°F, Gas Mark 9
CALORIES PER PORTION:
290 (1210 kilojoules)

For sousing a turkey you will need a large earthenware or terracotta casserole that can be used on direct heat, albeit with a heat diffusing mat if necessary. A metal pan or casserole is unsuitable due to its heat transmitting qualities – it gets too hot too quickly and cools down too fast. This method of cooking never fails to produce a succulent bird.

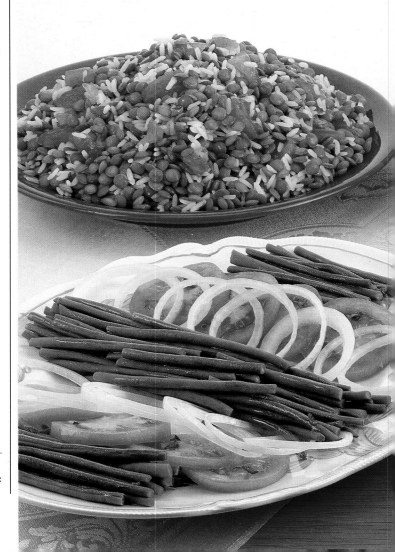

CLOCKWISE FROM TOP LEFT Lentil and tomato salad; Semi-soused turkey; Zucchini al forno; French bean salad

1. Place the turkey on a rack and lightly brown in the preheated oven for approximately 10 minutes.
2. Meanwhile heat the oil and lightly fry the onions and garlic.
3. Put the turkey, breast down, in a large casserole and snip the fresh herbs over. Sprinkle with salt, pepper and allspice and add the softened onions and garlic.
4. Combine all the liquids with the honey in a saucepan. Bring to the boil and pour over the bird. Cover the casserole, bring to the boil, turn down the heat and simmer for about 1½ hours. Turn the turkey over at least twice.

5. Remove from the heat but do not open the lid or turn the bird until completely cold. Leave to souse in the pot for at least 24 hours, turning the bird often.
6. To serve, remove the cold soused turkey from the pot and peel off the skin. Carve into thin slices, spooning the onions and juices over the meat to moisten.

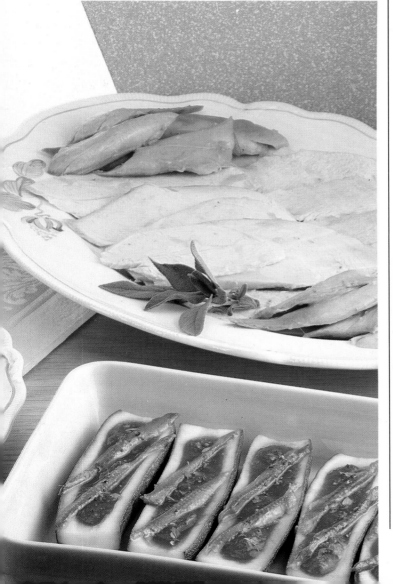

French Bean Salad

1 kg (2 lb) French beans, topped and tailed
1 garlic clove, peeled and lightly crushed
4 teaspoons green olive oil
1½ tablespoons lemon juice
salt
750 g (1½ lb) tomatoes, skinned and sliced
2 medium onions, peeled, sliced and separated into rings
freshly ground black pepper
2 teaspoons wine vinegar
chopped fresh oregano, marjoram or basil, to serve

PREPARATION TIME:
30 minutes, plus cooling
COOKING TIME:
8–10 minutes
CALORIES PER PORTION:
45 (190 kilojoules)

1. Trim the beans to equal lengths. Steam for about 8–10 minutes until just tender, then pour the water out of the saucepan below the steamer and put the beans immediately into the hot pan, adding the garlic clove, 2 teaspoons of the oil, the lemon juice and a sprinkling of salt. Replace the lid; shake well and set aside to cool.
2. When the beans are completely cold, discard the garlic and assemble the salad on a large flat platter. Starting at one end, arrange a row of beans, then a row of tomato, a row of onion on top of the tomatoes, then beans again, and so on.
3. Sprinkle everything lightly with salt and pepper and drizzle the remaining oil and the vinegar over the tomatoes and onions only. Sprinkle the platter with chopped oregano and serve.

Lentil and Tomato Salad

275 g (10 oz) green lentils, washed
175 g (6 oz) long-grain rice
6 large tomatoes, peeled, seeded and chopped
1 tablespoon olive oil
2 garlic cloves, peeled and finely chopped
1 teaspoon cumin seed
1 teaspoon black mustard seed
1 tablespoon vinegar
2 teaspoons lemon juice
salt
pepper

PREPARATION TIME:
15 minutes
COOKING TIME:
10–15 minutes
CALORIES PER PORTION:
190 (795 kilojoules)

1. Put the lentils in a large saucepan with plenty of cold water. Do not add salt. Bring to the boil, cover and simmer gently for about 10–12 minutes. If done to your liking, strain and set aside.
2. Bring a pan of water to the boil and add the rice, simmer for 10–12 minutes then drain, and set aside.
3. Combine the lentils, rice and tomatoes in a serving bowl. Heat the oil in a frying pan and fry the garlic, cumin and mustard seed until the garlic is almost burnt; tip over the lentil mixture at once.
4. Sprinkle over the vinegar and lemon juice, season with salt and pepper and mix thoroughly.

Menu continues over page

Seasonal Berries

225 g (8 oz) blackcurrants,
  topped and tailed
450 g (1 lb) strawberries,
  hulled and quartered or
  halved, according to size
450 g (1 lb) raspberries,
  hulled
225 g (8 oz) cultivated
  blackberries, topped and
  tailed
225 g (8 oz) loganberries,
  hulled
300 ml (½ pint) rosé wine
½ teaspoon ground allspice

PREPARATION TIME:
10 minutes
COOKING TIME:
5 minutes, plus marinating
CALORIES PER PORTION:
40 (170 kilojoules)

1. Combine all the berries
in a serving bowl.
2. In a saucepan heat the
wine to boiling point, add
the allspice and pour over
the fruit at once.
3. Cool and stand at room
temperature for 4–6
hours.

Sparkling Lime

5–6 fresh limes, squeezed and
  strained
1.2 litres (2 pints) sparkling
  mineral water
1 teaspoon Angostura bitters
5 tablespoons brandy
  (optional)

PREPARATION TIME:
3 minutes, plus chilling
CALORIES PER PORTION:
10 (40 kilojoules)

If you choose not to
include brandy this drink
has a sharp and very
refreshing taste which you
may feel needs
sweetening. If necessary,
add artificial sweetener to
taste.

1. Chill the lime juice and
mineral water separately.
2. Combine with the other
ingredients and serve in
tall glasses.

BELOW, FROM TOP Sparkling lime;
Seasonal berries

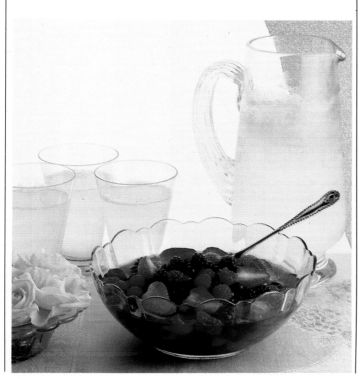

JUNE

Hors d'oeuvres and Light Meals

Peperonata with Wholemeal Noodles

Peperonata is a classic
summer dish, combining
the best of the summer
produce – peppers, fresh
tomatoes and fresh basil.
Use fresh wholemeal
noodles if you can find
them, these will take about
8–10 minutes to cook.

3 tablespoons olive oil
2 large onions, peeled and
  thinly sliced
1 large garlic clove, peeled
  and crushed
2 red peppers, seeded and cut
  into strips
2 green peppers, seeded and
  cut into strips
450 g (1 lb) tomatoes,
  skinned, seeded and chopped
1 tablespoon chopped fresh
  basil
salt
freshly ground black pepper
175 g (6 oz) wholemeal
  noodles
sprigs of fresh basil, to
  garnish (optional)

PREPARATION TIME:
20–25 minutes
COOKING TIME:
20 minutes
CALORIES PER PORTION:
315 (1320 kilojoules)

1. Heat 2 tablespoons olive
oil in a deep frying pan.
Add the onions and garlic
and cook very gently until
the onions soften.
2. Add the peppers,
tomatoes, basil and salt
and pepper to taste. Cover
and cook gently for 10
minutes.
3. Remove the lid from the
pan and cook over a fairly
high heat until most of the
moisture has evaporated.
Keep warm.
4. Meanwhile cook the
noodles in plenty of boiling
salted water until just
tender.
5. Drain the noodles
thoroughly and toss in the
remaining olive oil; add
salt and pepper to taste.
6. Divide the noodles
among 4 serving plates and
spoon the hot peperonata
over the top.
7. Garnish with sprigs of
fresh basil and serve
immediately, as a light
main course with a salad.

Globe Artichokes with Yogurt Dressing

150 ml (¼ pint) plain
  unsweetened yogurt
½ lemon
1 garlic clove, peeled and
  crushed
1 tablespoon chopped chives
½ red pepper, seeded and
  finely chopped
salt
freshly ground black pepper
4 globe artichokes

PREPARATION TIME:
30 minutes, plus chilling
COOKING TIME:
30 minutes
CALORIES PER PORTION:
25 (105 kilojoules)

1. To make the dressing,
mix the yogurt with the
finely grated rind of the ½
lemon, garlic, chives and
red pepper; add salt and
pepper to taste.
2. Chill the yogurt dressing
very thoroughly.
3. Trim off the stem from
the base of each globe
artichoke. Cut off the top
of each artichoke about
2 cm (¾ inch) down.
4. Rub the cut surfaces of
the artichoke with the
derinded ½ lemon.
5. Lower the prepared
globe artichokes into a
large pan of boiling water;
bring back to the boil, and
cook covered for about 30
minutes, until the
artichokes are tender. (Pull
off one leaf; nibble the end
and if it is tender then the
artichoke is cooked.)
6. Leave the artichokes
upside-down on a clean
teatowel until thoroughly
drained.
7. Stand each artichoke
upright on a small serving
plate, and serve the chilled
yogurt dressing in a
separate bowl.

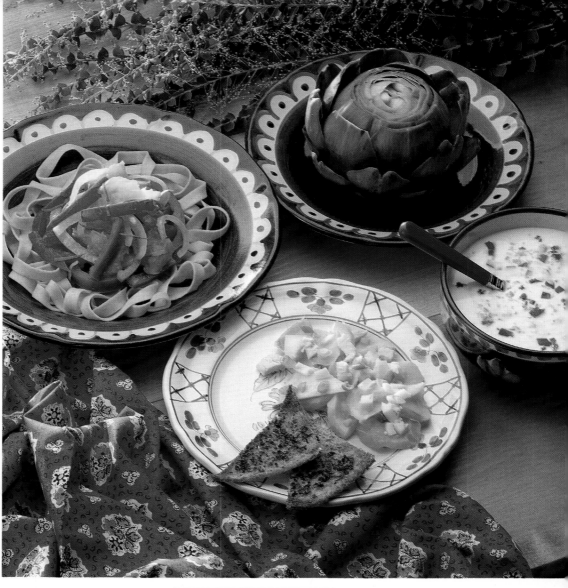

Flaked Haddock with Parsleyed Melba Toast

350 g (12 oz) smoked haddock
  fillet
grated rind of ½ lemon
150 ml (¼ pint) dry white
  wine
pinch of ground nutmeg
salt
freshly ground black pepper
1 hard-boiled egg, shelled and
  chopped
2 thin spring onions, finely
  sliced
fennel leaves or fresh parsley,
  to garnish (optional)
Melba toast:
2 thin slices wholemeal bread
  (from a cut loaf)
15 g (½ oz) low fat spread
finely chopped parsley

PREPARATION TIME:
25 minutes
COOKING TIME:
15 minutes
CALORIES PER PORTION:
108 (750 kilojoules)

1. Put the haddock into a
shallow pan with the
lemon rind, white wine,
nutmeg and salt and
pepper to taste.
2. Cover and cook gently
until the fish is just tender
– about 10 minutes.
3. Skin the haddock and
remove any stray bones;
flake the flesh.
4. Mix the fish with the
hard-boiled egg and spring
onions and adjust
seasoning to taste. Keep
warm.
5. Toast the slices of
wholemeal bread on both
sides then remove the

crusts and cut each slice in
half horizontally, using a
very sharp knife.
6. Spread the untoasted
surfaces with *a little* low fat
spread and sprinkle
generously with chopped
parsley.
7. Place the slices under a
preheated grill, just long
enough to curl the toast
without burning it.
8. Spoon the warm
smoked haddock mixture
on to small plates and
garnish with fennel leaves
or parsley, if using.
9. Serve immediately with
the freshly made melba
toast.

ABOVE, CLOCKWISE FROM LEFT
Peperonata with wholemeal noodles;
Globe artichokes with yogurt dressing;
Flaked haddock with parsleyed melba
toast

JUNE

Main Courses

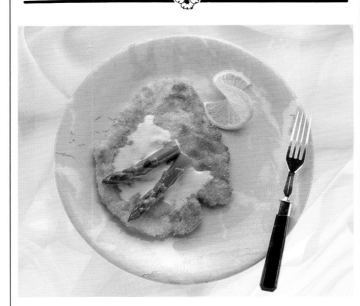

Turkey Escalopes with Asparagus

4 turkey escalopes, about
  150 g (5 oz) each, beaten flat
1 tablespoon plain flour
3 tablespoons fine dry
  breadcrumbs
finely grated rind of 1 lemon
salt
freshly ground black pepper
1 egg, beaten
25 g (1 oz) butter
2 tablespoons olive oil
Sauce:
4 tablespoons lemon juice
2 tablespoons chicken stock
1 egg yolk
To garnish:
8–12 cooked asparagus tips
4 lemon twists

PREPARATION TIME:
15 minutes
COOKING TIME:
12 minutes
CALORIES PER PORTION:
350 (1460 kilojoules)

1. Dust the turkey escalopes with flour.
2. Mix the breadcrumbs with the lemon rind and salt and pepper to taste.
3. Dip the escalopes into beaten egg and then coat evenly with the seasoned breadcrumbs.
4. Heat the butter and oil in a large shallow pan and fry the turkey escalopes for about 4 minutes on each side. Drain and keep warm.
5. For the sauce, put the lemon juice into a small pan with the stock and bring to the boil. Place the egg yolk in a basin and gradually whisk in the lemon and stock. Return the mixture to the pan and stir over a gentle heat until thickened.
6. Arrange the cooked escalopes on a serving dish; spoon a pool of sauce on top of each and garnish with asparagus tips and a twist of lemon.

Fish Kebabs Madras

4 tablespoons plain
  unsweetened yogurt
3 tablespoons lime juice
1 garlic clove, peeled and
  crushed
1 teaspoon curry powder
6 drops Tabasco sauce
1 thin slice fresh ginger, finely
  chopped
salt
freshly ground black pepper
500 g (1 lb 2 oz) monkfish or
  other firm white fish, cut into
  2.5 cm (1 inch) cubes
12 large peeled prawns
12 shelled mussels
To garnish:
1 tablespoon roughly chopped
  fresh coriander
thin lime wedges

PREPARATION TIME:
15 minutes, plus chilling
COOKING TIME:
about 6 minutes
CALORIES PER PORTION:
160 (670 kilojoules)

1. Mix the yogurt with the lime juice, garlic, curry powder, Tabasco, chopped ginger and salt and pepper.
2. Stir the fish, prawns and mussels lightly into the spiced yogurt mixture; cover and chill for 4 hours.
3. Thread the pieces of fish, prawns and mussels alternately on to 4 kebab skewers; brush off any excess yogurt mixture.
4. Place the kebabs on a lightly greased baking sheet under a preheated grill; grill for about 6 minutes until the fish is just tender, brushing with extra yogurt marinade.
5. Arrange the kebabs on a platter, sprinkle with coriander and serve with wedges of lime.

ABOVE Turkey escalopes with asparagus RIGHT, FROM TOP Fish kebabs Madras; Noodles with fresh beans, peas and tarragon

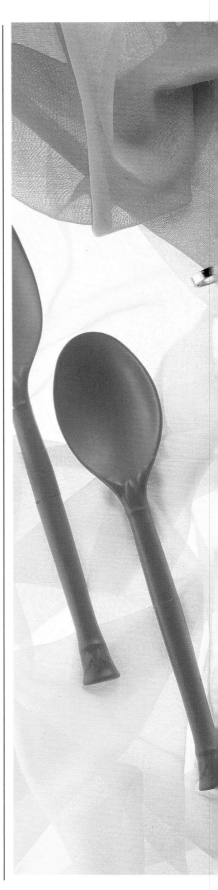

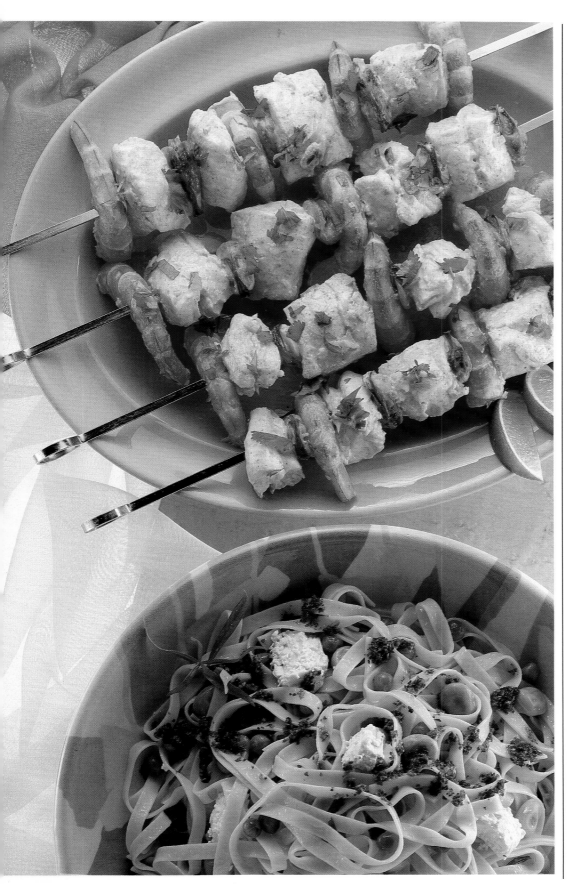

Noodles with Fresh Beans, Peas and Tarragon

1 bunch watercress, washed
  and roughly chopped
1 garlic clove, peeled
200 ml (⅓ pint) chicken stock
salt
freshly ground black pepper
175 g (6 oz) shelled fresh peas
175 g (6 oz) shelled fresh
  broad beans
350 g (12 oz) tagliatelle
  noodles
50 g (2 oz) cream cheese, cut
  into small pieces
1 tablespoon chopped fresh
  tarragon
small sprigs of fresh tarragon,
  to garnish

PREPARATION TIME:
25 minutes
COOKING TIME:
about 10 minutes
CALORIES PER PORTION:
440 (1840 kilojoules)

1. Put the watercress, garlic, chicken stock and salt and pepper to taste into the liquidizer; blend until smooth.
2. Put the shelled peas and broad beans into a steamer (or a colander standing over a pan of simmering water) and steam until just tender.
3. Meanwhile cook the noodles in plenty of boiling salted water until tender.
4. Drain the noodles thoroughly and stir in the cream cheese and chopped tarragon; toss together with the steamed peas and broad beans and adjust seasoning to taste.
5. Transfer to a serving dish and spoon over the prepared watercress sauce. Garnish with sprigs of fresh tarragon and serve immediately.

JUNE

Puddings

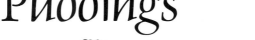

Peach Granita

350 g (12 oz) fresh ripe
 peaches
150 ml (¼ pint) dry white
 wine
150 ml (¼ pint) fresh orange
 juice
2 egg whites

PREPARATION TIME:
20–25 minutes, plus freezing
COOKING TIME:
5 minutes
CALORIES PER PORTION:
80 (335 kilojoules)

1. Nick the stalk end of
each peach; plunge into a
bowl of boiling water for
45 seconds, then slide off
the skins. Halve the fruit,
removing the stones, and

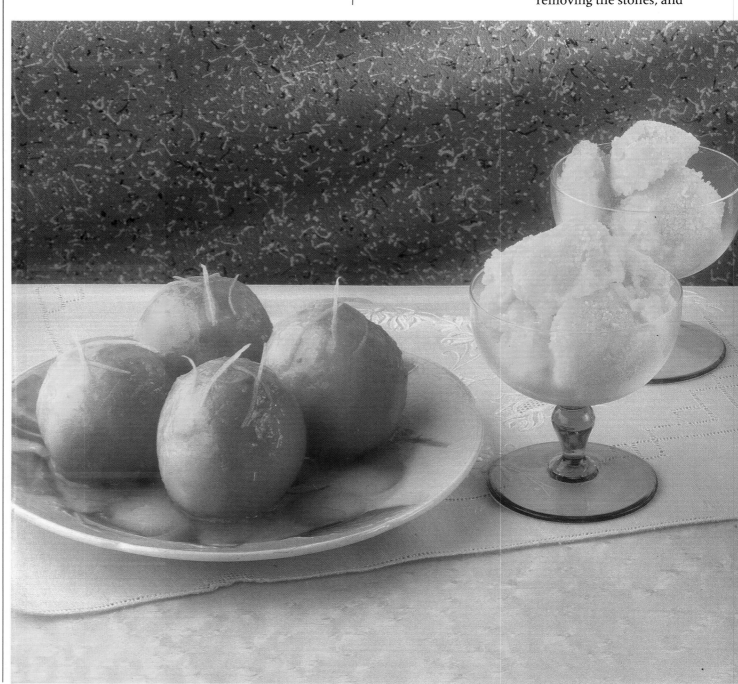

chop the flesh roughly.
2. Put the peach flesh into a pan with the white wine and orange juice. (If you have a very sweet tooth, add a little artificial sweetener.) Simmer gently for 5 minutes.
3. Blend the peaches and the liquid in the liquidizer until smooth. Cool.
4. Put into a shallow container; freeze until the granita is 'slushy' around the edges, then tip into a bowl and break up the ice crystals.
5. Whisk the egg whites until stiff but not dry; fold lightly but thoroughly into the partly-frozen granita. Return to the container and re-freeze until firm.

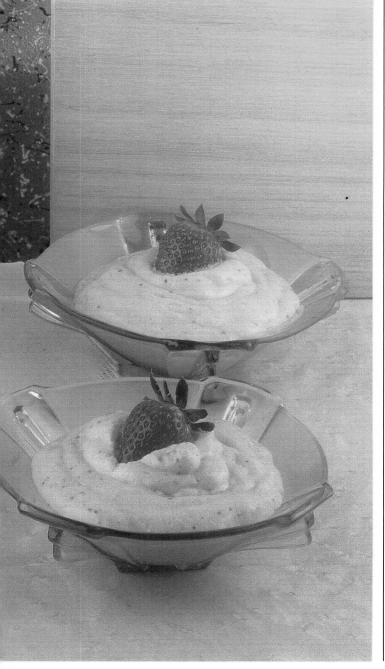

Marinated Nectarines

4 large ripe nectarines
1 lemon
1 large orange
200 ml (⅓ pint) water
4 tablespoons dry vermouth

PREPARATION TIME:
25–30 minutes, plus chilling
CALORIES PER PORTION:
75 (315 kilojoules)

1. Nick the stalk end of each nectarine; plunge into a bowl of boiling water for 45 seconds, then slide off the skins.
2. Pare the skin from the lemon and cut into matchstick strips. Squeeze the lemon juice into a large bowl and fill up with iced water. Put the prepared nectarines into the lemon water.
3. Peel the orange thinly, removing all the pith; chop the flesh into pieces, discarding any pips. Cut the orange peel into matchstick strips.
4. Put the orange flesh into the liquidizer with the water and vermouth; blend until smooth.
5. Lift the nectarines out of the lemon water and drain.
6. Put the nectarines into a shallow dish and spoon over the prepared orange and vermouth sauce. Cover and chill for 2 hours. (No longer, otherwise the nectarines are likely to discolour.)
7. Sprinkle with the strips of lemon and orange peel and serve immediately.

Strawberry and Orange Chiffon

350 g (12 oz) ripe strawberries
6 tablespoons orange juice
finely grated rind of ½ orange
1 tablespoon honey
2 eggs, separated
2 teaspoons powdered gelatine
2 tablespoons water
4 tablespoons plain unsweetened yogurt

PREPARATION TIME:
about 40 minutes, plus chilling
CALORIES PER PORTION:
120 (505 kilojoules)

1. Reserve 4 whole strawberries for decoration.
2. Put the remaining strawberries into the liquidizer and blend until smooth.
3. Put the orange juice and rind, honey and egg yolks into a bowl; whisk until thick, light and creamy.
4. Put the gelatine and the water in a heatproof bowl and stand in a saucepan of hot water. Stir until the gelatine has dissolved.
5. Combine the strawberry purée and whisked egg yolk mixture, then stir in the dissolved gelatine and the yogurt.
6. Whisk the egg whites until stiff but not dry; as soon as the strawberry mixture is on the point of setting, fold in the whites lightly but thoroughly.
7. Spoon into glass dessert dishes and chill for 2–3 hours.
8. Decorate each dessert with one of the reserved whole strawberries and serve.

FROM THE LEFT Marinated nectarines; Peach granita; Strawberry and orange chiffon

JUNE

Dinner Party for Six

A simple and delicious summertime menu. If necessary the soup may be prepared in advance and served cold, but you will need to taste and adjust the seasoning just before serving as chilling may dull the flavour slightly.

Marrow and Dill Soup

1 kg (2 lb) marrow, peeled, seeded and grated
salt
½ tablespoon oil
½ tablespoon plain flour
1 tablespoon mild French mustard
1 tablespoon dried dill
900 ml (1½ pints) chicken stock
1 tablespoon lemon juice
1 teaspoon sugar (optional)
paprika, to serve

PREPARATION TIME:
10 minutes, plus standing
COOKING TIME:
20 minutes
CALORIES PER PORTION:
60 (250 kilojoules)

1. Place the marrow in a colander, sprinkle a little salt over and leave to stand for 20 minutes.
2. Heat the oil in a large saucepan, put in the marrow and sprinkle with the flour. Stir well then cook for 1 minute, stirring all the time.
3. Add the mustard and half the dill, stir, then pour the stock in slowly, still stirring. Cover and simmer very gently for 15–20 minutes, do not allow to boil vigorously.
4. For a smooth textured soup, cool slightly then blend in a liquidizer. Taste and adjust the seasoning, adding lemon juice and sugar as necessary. Stir in the remaining dill.
5. Pour into warmed soup bowls, sprinkle a little paprika over each portion and serve. For a richer soup 1 teaspoonful of soured cream may be placed in the bottom of each bowl before the soup is poured in. This will increase the calories per portion to 90 (380 kilojoules).

Sweet and Sour Fish

2 teaspoons oil
3 garlic cloves, peeled and finely chopped
2 red peppers, seeded and cut into thin strips
1 kg (2 lb) huss or monkfish, cut into 2.5 cm (1 inch) cubes
4 fresh tomatoes, skinned and chopped
1 tablespoon tomato, peach or mango chutney
2 tablespoons light soy sauce
2 teaspoons vinegar
100 g (4 oz) walnut pieces
1 teaspoon grated fresh ginger

PREPARATION TIME:
10 minutes
COOKING TIME:
7–10 minutes
CALORIES PER PORTION:
300 (1260 kilojoules)

1. Heat the oil in a large non-stick frying pan or wok. Fry the garlic and red pepper.
2. Add the fish to the pan and stir gently; add the tomatoes, chutney, soy sauce and vinegar.
3. Add the walnuts and grated ginger to the fish. Stir gently then cover and cook for about 3 minutes. Taste and adjust seasoning.
4. Serve with fusilli (pasta twists) and a salad.

Raspberry and Yogurt Ice Cream

225 g (8 oz) fresh raspberries
50 g (2 oz) icing sugar
2 tablespoons clear honey
2 tablespoons lemon juice
900 ml (1½ pints) plain unsweetened yogurt
sprigs of fresh salad burnet (if available), to garnish

PREPARATION TIME:
10 minutes, plus freezing
CALORIES PER PORTION:
110 (460 kilojoules)

Ice cream is easy to make, but to be really successful it needs to freeze fast and be churned all the time if possible, ideally in an ice cream machine, or stirred to break up the ice crystals at regular intervals. The more agitation it has, the lighter the end result.

1. Set the refrigerator at its lowest temperature.
2. Liquidize the raspberries then push them through a sieve. Add all the other ingredients, stir well and freeze as fast as possible (see above) in the freezing compartment of the refrigerator or in the freezer.
3. Scoop the ice cream into glasses and decorate each serving with a sprig of salad burnet.

CLOCKWISE FROM BOTTOM RIGHT
Sweet and sour fish, served with pasta and green salad; Raspberry and yogurt ice cream; Marrow and dill soup

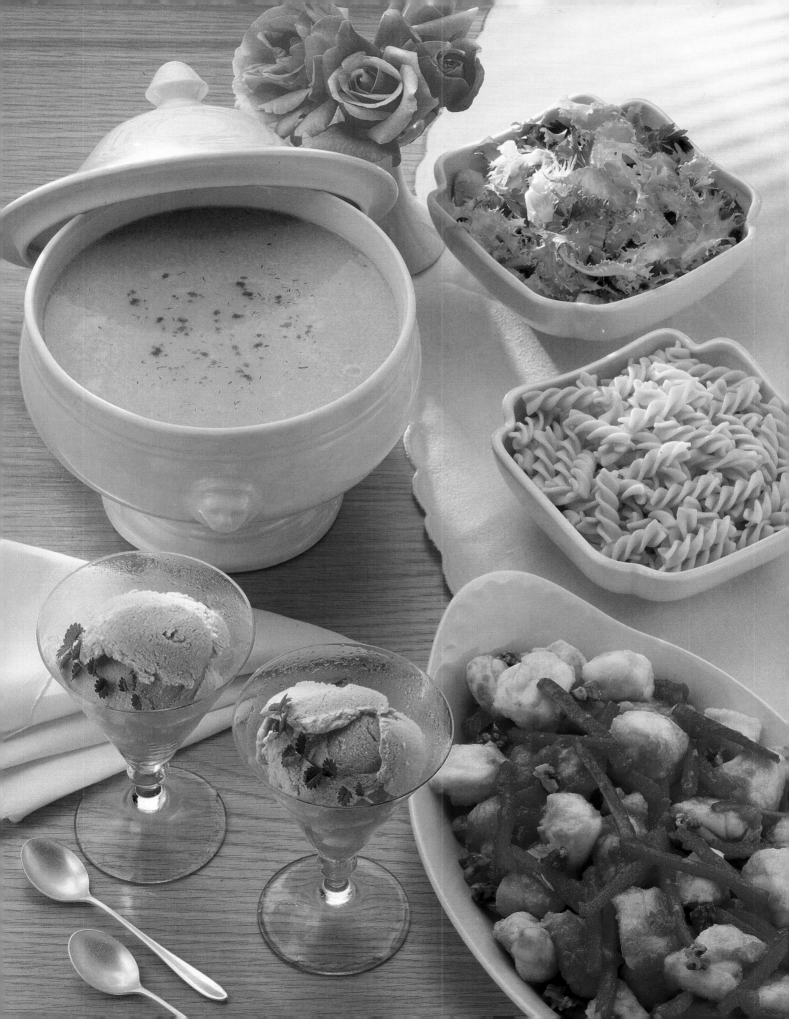

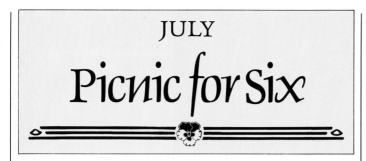

JULY
Picnic for Six

There is no reason why a picnic should be a collection of tired sandwiches. A stylish meal laid out on a cloth on the ground in idyllic surroundings is a thoroughly enjoyable event, and this menu is as easy to prepare, pack and serve as a conventional picnic.

Picnic Pizza

Bread base:
225 g (8 oz) strong white
    plain flour
½ teaspoon salt
65 ml (2½ fl oz) skimmed
    milk, warmed
65 ml (2½ fl oz) warm water
1 teaspoon dried yeast
½ teaspoon soft brown sugar
Topping:
2 tablespoons tomato purée
1 large garlic clove, peeled
    and finely sliced
3 tomatoes, skinned and
    thinly sliced
5 small fresh sardines, filleted
salt
freshly ground black pepper
6 mushrooms, thinly sliced
1 red pepper, cored, seeded
    and thinly sliced
5 anchovy fillets, halved
5 black olives, whole or sliced
1 tablespoon finely chopped
    fresh parsley
1 tablespoon green olive oil

PREPARATION TIME:
45 minutes, plus proving
COOKING TIME:
25 minutes
OVEN TEMPERATURE:
220°C, 425°F, Gas Mark 7
CALORIES PER PORTION:
280 (1180 kilojoules)

1. Sift the flour with the salt. Combine the milk with the water, sprinkle the dried yeast over the liquids and whisk in the sugar. Leave in a warm place for 30 minutes until frothy.
2. Make a well in the centre of the flour and pour in the liquid. Mix well together, then turn out on to a floured surface and knead thoroughly for 8–10 minutes.
3. Place the dough in a lightly oiled polythene bag and set in a bowl in a warm place to rise until doubled in size (about 1 hour).
4. Turn the dough on to a floured surface and knead again. Roll it into a circle 30 cm (12 inches) in diameter and place on an oiled and floured baking tray.
5. Spread the tomato purée over the dough and sprinkle with garlic. Arrange the tomato on top.
6. Sprinkle the sardines with salt and pepper and arrange on the pizza with the mushroom and red pepper slices, halved anchovy fillets and olives. Sprinkle with parsley and oil.
8. Bake in a preheated oven for approximately 25 minutes. Cool.

Multi-Coloured Bean Salad

1 × 225 g (8 oz) can chick
    peas, drained
1 × 225 g (8 oz) can red
    kidney beans, drained
1 × 225 g (8 oz) can white
    kidney beans, drained
225 g (8 oz) cooked French
    beans, chopped into 2.5 cm
    (1 inch) lengths
1 red pepper, cored, seeded
    and finely sliced
1 bunch spring onions,
    chopped
2 garlic cloves, peeled
½ teaspoon salt
2 tablespoons tahini
1 tablespoon lemon juice
1 tablespoon soy sauce
2 tablespoons water
1 tablespoon chopped fresh
    parsley or coriander

PREPARATION TIME:
15 minutes plus marinating
CALORIES PER PORTION:
325 (1365 kilojoules)

1. Rinse all the canned beans. Combine with the French beans, red pepper and spring onions in a deep serving bowl.
2. Crush the garlic with the salt and combine the tahini, lemon juice, soy sauce and water. If the dressing is too thick add a little more water. Stir the dressing into the beans and sprinkle the parsley over.
3. Leave to marinate for 2 hours before serving.

FROM THE RIGHT Picnic pizza; Summer cup; Melon surprise; Summer terrine; Multi-coloured bean salad

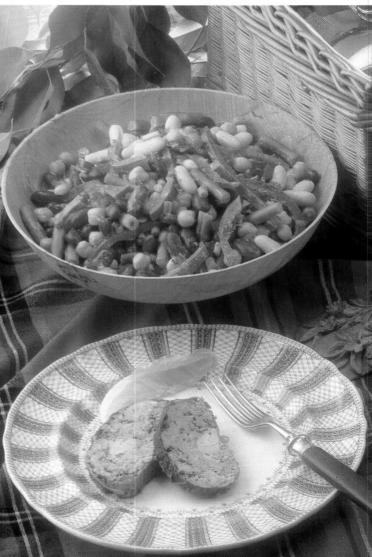

Summer Terrine

750 g (1½ lb) minced veal
275 g (10 oz) calves' liver,
  minced
3 garlic cloves, peeled and
  finely chopped
1 teaspoon chopped fresh
  rosemary
1 tablespoon puréed cooked
  spinach
1 tablespoon lemon juice
salt
freshly ground black pepper
10–12 undamaged large
  lettuce leaves
4 tablespoons white wine
1 teaspoon oil

PREPARATION TIME:
25–30 minutes
COOKING TIME:
1½ hours
OVEN TEMPERATURE:
180°C, 350°F, Gas Mark 4
CALORIES PER PORTION:
220 (920 kilojoules)

1. Mix the meats together
with the garlic, rosemary,
spinach and lemon juice.
Season with plenty of salt
and freshly ground black
pepper then knead lightly.
2. Blanch the lettuce leaves
for 1 minute in boiling
water, then drop them into
cold water, drain them and
lay them out to dry on
clean teatowels.
3. Lay a sheet of non-stick
silicone paper on the work
top and arrange 5–6
lettuce leaves in a row,
slightly overlapping, on
top. Arrange the other
leaves in another row next
to the first so that the stalk
ends overlap.
4. Spoon the meat mixture
down the centre of the
leaves. Compress it with
your hands into a large
sausage shape, then fold
over the leaves so they
meet and overlap on top.
5. Carefully transfer the
roll, on the silicone paper,
to an earthenware baking
dish. Pour the wine over
and, using a pastry brush,
paint the exposed leaves
with the oil. Cover with
more silicone paper, cover
with a lid or foil and bake
in a preheated oven for 1½
hours. Allow to cool before
uncovering.

Melon Surprise

6 small Gallia melons, about
  350 g (12 oz) each
2 medium mangoes
4 kiwi fruits
6 teaspoons Cointreau

PREPARATION TIME:
20 minutes
CALORIES PER PORTION:
110 (460 kilojoules)

1. Slice off the tops of the
melons and scoop out the
seeds, pulp and all the
flesh, without damaging
the shell. Do not remove
the flesh from the lids.
2. Slice the melon flesh
into thin strips.
3. Peel the mangoes and
kiwi fruits. Cut the
mangoes into strips, slice
and halve the kiwis.
Combine all the fruit.
4. Put 1 teaspoon of
Cointreau in each melon,
spoon in the fruit mixture
and replace the lids.

Summer Cup

450 g (1 lb) raspberries
1 tablespoon water
600 ml (1 pint) sparkling
  mineral water
1 bottle sparkling white wine
2 tablespoons Cassis

PREPARATION TIME:
5 minutes, plus chilling overnight
COOKING TIME:
5 minutes
CALORIES PER PORTION:
60 (250 kilojoules)

1. Crush the raspberries
and put them in a
saucepan with the
tablespoon of water; bring
to boiling point and
simmer for 3 minutes.
Cool, then combine with
the other ingredients and
place in an airtight
container. Refrigerate
overnight.
2. Strain the cup and place
in a chilled vacuum flask.

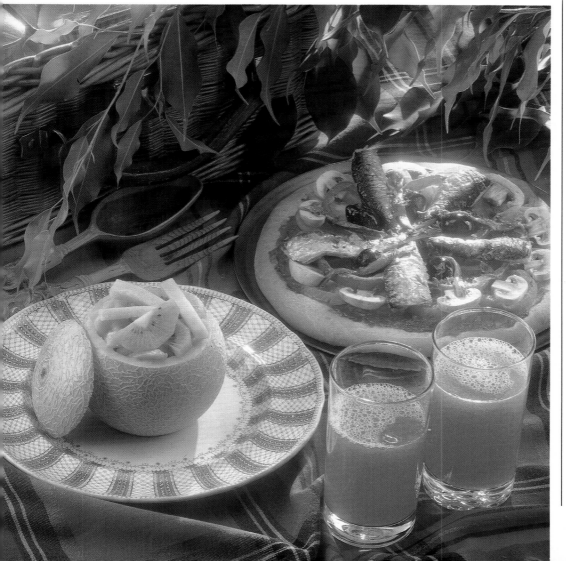

Hors d'oeuvres and Light Meals

Gazpacho

450 g (1 lb) tomatoes,
  skinned, seeded and chopped
1 green pepper, seeded and
  roughly chopped
1 red pepper, seeded and
  roughly chopped
1 small onion, peeled and
  roughly chopped
1 large garlic clove, peeled
  and chopped
about 450 ml (¾ pint)
  chicken stock
salt
freshly ground black pepper
1 tablespoon lemon juice
  (optional)
To garnish:
ice cubes
cucumber slices
1 tablespoon finely chopped
  red pepper

PREPARATION TIME:
about 25 minutes, plus chilling
CALORIES PER PORTION:
120 (500 kilojoules)

1. Put the tomatoes,
peppers, onion, garlic and
chicken stock into the
liquidizer; blend until
fairly smooth.
2. Pour the blended soup
into a bowl and season to
taste, adding the lemon
juice if necessary. Cover
the soup and chill for at
least 3 hours.
3. Ladle the chilled soup
into soup bowls; add an ice
cube to each one, and float
cucumber slices sprinkled
with a little chopped red
pepper on top.

Oeufs en Gelée

4 eggs
1 × 5 cm (2 inch) piece
  cucumber, peeled, seeded
  and finely chopped
1 tablespoon chopped chives
1 teaspoon chopped fresh
  tarragon
400 ml (⅔ pint) consommé
  (unchilled)
To garnish:
sprigs fresh tarragon
4 slices brown bread, cut into
  thin fingers and lightly
  spread with butter

PREPARATION TIME:
about 20 minutes, plus chilling
COOKING TIME:
3 minutes
CALORIES PER PORTION:
150 (630 kilojoules)

1. Lower the eggs carefully
into a pan of boiling water,
and boil for exactly 3
minutes (no longer). Allow
to cool slightly, then
carefully remove the
shells.
2. Place the eggs into 4
small cocotte dishes with
the cucumber, and add a
sprinkling of chopped
chives and tarragon; top
up each dish with liquid
consommé. (It should
cover the eggs.)
3.Chill until the consommé
has set – about 3 hours.
4. Garnish each cocotte
dish with a sprig of
tarragon, and serve the
Oeufs en gelée with fingers
of brown bread and butter.

Prawn and Curd Cheese Mousses

225 g (8 oz) sieved cottage or
  low fat curd cheese
150 ml (¼ pint) plain
  unsweetened yogurt
150 ml (¼ pint) chicken stock
2 tablespoons dry white wine
3 teaspoons powdered gelatine
1 tablespoon chopped fresh
  dill
salt
freshly ground black pepper
100 g (4 oz) peeled prawns,
  chopped
dill sprigs, to garnish
Sauce:
3 tablespoons low calorie
  mayonnaise
½–1 tablespoon lemon juice
1 tablespoon dry white wine

PREPARATION TIME:
30 minutes, plus chilling
CALORIES PER PORTION:
140 (590 kilojoules)

1. Mix the cottage cheese
with the yogurt and
chicken stock; beat until
quite smooth.
2. Put the wine and
gelatine into a small bowl;
stand in a pan of hot water
and stir until the gelatine
has dissolved.
3. Stir the gelatine into the
cheese mixture, and add
the chopped dill, salt and
pepper to taste and the
chopped prawns.
4. Spoon the prepared
mixture into 4 or 8 lightly
greased individual moulds
(depending on size); chill
until set, about 3 hours.
5. For the sauce, mix the
mayonnaise, lemon juice
and white wine together,
adding salt and pepper.
6. Unmould 1 or 2 set
mousses on to 4 small
plates, spoon on some
sauce and garnish with a
sprig of dill.

FROM THE LEFT Oeufs en gelée;
Gazpacho; Prawn and curd cheese
mousses

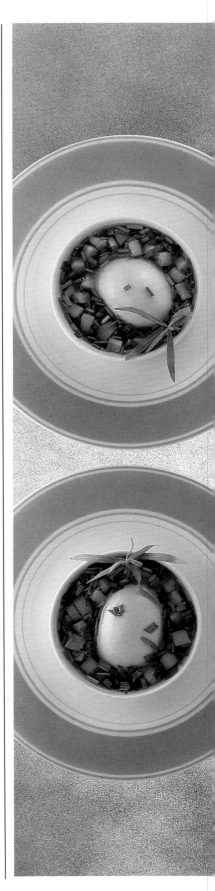

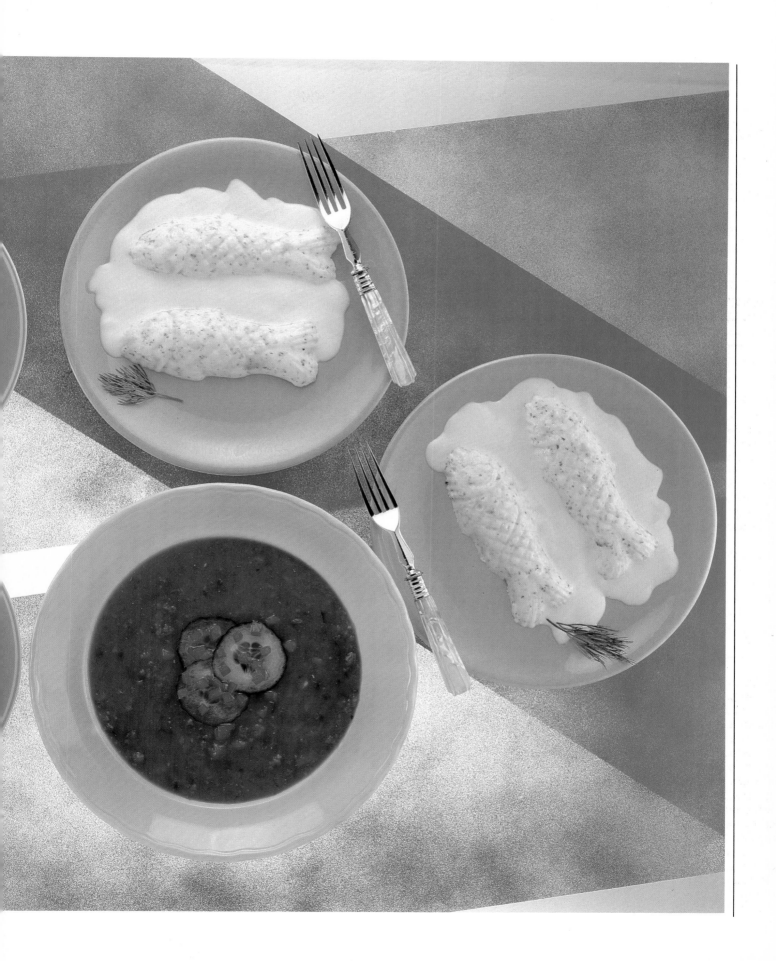

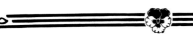

JULY

Main Courses

Two Cheese Lasagne

300 ml (½ pint) skimmed
  milk
1 bay leaf
1 small onion stuck with
  4 cloves
20 g (¾ oz) butter
20 g (¾ oz) plain flour
salt
freshly ground black pepper
225 g (8 oz) runner beans,
  sliced
150 g (5 oz) green or
  wholemeal quick-cook
  lasagne
225 g (8 oz) cottage cheese,
  sieved
2 tablespoons chopped parsley
1 garlic clove, peeled and
  crushed
150 ml (¼ pint) plain
  unsweetened yogurt
1 egg
3 tablespoons grated
  Parmesan cheese

PREPARATION TIME:
20 minutes
COOKING TIME:
about 55 minutes
OVEN TEMPERATURE:
190°C, 375°F, Gas Mark 5
CALORIES PER PORTION:
400 (1675 kilojoules)

1. Put the skimmed milk
into a pan with the bay leaf
and onion. Bring to the
boil and leave to stand, off
the heat, for 15 minutes.
2. Heat the butter in a pan
and stir in the flour; cook
for 1 minute. Gradually stir
in the strained milk and
stir over a moderate heat
until thickened. Add salt
and pepper to taste.

3. Cook the beans in a
small amount of boiling
water until almost tender –
do not overcook – then
drain and save the liquid.
4. Put one-third of the
lasagne into a lightly
greased ovenproof dish;
thin the white sauce with a
little of the bean cooking
liquid, and spoon half the
sauce over the lasagne.
5. Top with the cooked
green beans, and then with
a second layer of dry
lasagne.
6. Mix the cottage cheese
with the parsley and garlic.
Put a layer of the cottage
cheese mixture over the
lasagne and top with the
remaining sauce. Arrange
the remaining sheets of
lasagne on the top.
7. Beat the yogurt with the
egg, Parmesan cheese and
salt and pepper to taste;
spoon over the top of the
lasagne.
8. Bake in the oven for
about 45 minutes until
golden; serve piping hot.

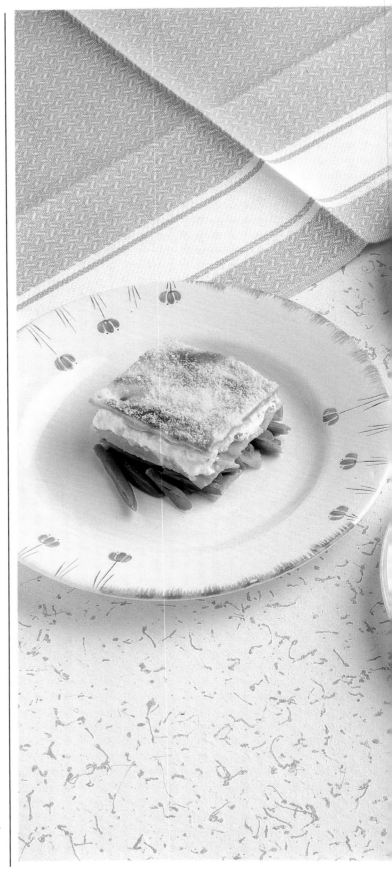

CLOCKWISE FROM LEFT Two cheese
lasagne; Plaice with courgette and
lemon sauce; Skewered lamb

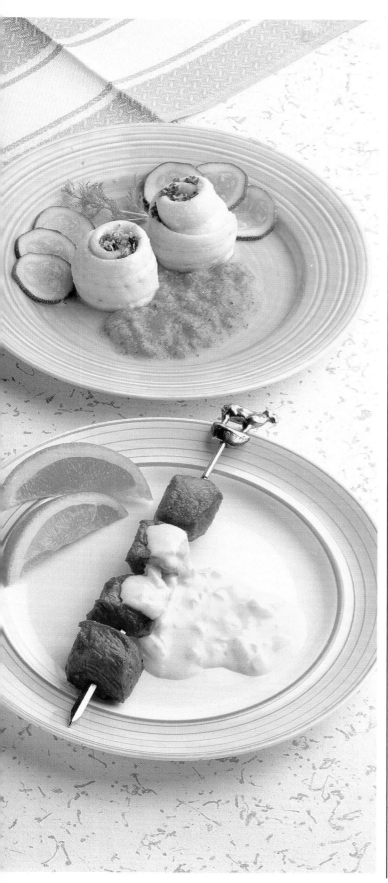

Plaice with Courgette and Lemon Sauce

8 small plaice fillets, about
  65 g (2½ oz) each, skinned
salt
freshly ground black pepper
finely grated rind of ½ lemon
1 tablespoon finely chopped
  parsley
300 ml (½ pint) skimmed
  milk
Sauce:
350 g (12 oz) courgettes
300 ml (½ pint) chicken stock
grated rind of ½ lemon
1 garlic clove, peeled and
  chopped
dill sprigs, to garnish

PREPARATION TIME:
25–30 minutes
COOKING TIME:
about 15 minutes
CALORIES PER PORTION:
160 (670 kilojoules)

1. Spread out the plaice
fillets skinned sides
uppermost. Sprinkle with
salt and pepper to taste,
lemon rind and parsley,
and roll each one up.
2. For the sauce, chop the
courgettes and cook
together with the stock,
lemon rind and garlic until
just tender.
3. Blend the cooked
courgettes and their liquid
until smooth.
4. Put the rolled plaice
fillets into a shallow pan;
add the milk and salt and
pepper to taste. Poach the
fish gently until it is just
tender, about 8–10
minutes, then drain,
reserving the liquid. Put on
a warm serving dish.
5. Heat the courgette purée
in a pan with sufficient of
the fish cooking liquid to
give a fairly slack sauce.
6. Spoon the prepared
courgette and lemon sauce
around the rolled fish
fillets and garnish with dill.
Serve with courgettes.

Skewered Lamb

450 g (1 lb) lamb fillet, cut
  into 2.5 cm (1 inch) cubes
¼ teaspoon crushed black
  peppercorns
salt
150 ml (¼ pint) white wine
coarsely grated rind of
  ½ orange
pinch of ground cinnamon
1 small onion, thinly sliced
Sauce:
1 small onion, finely chopped
1 tablespoon olive oil
pinch of saffron strands
1 egg yolk
2 tablespoons plain
  unsweetened yogurt
juice of ½ orange
1 teaspoon cornflour
artificial sweetener, to taste

PREPARATION TIME:
about 30 minutes, plus chilling
COOKING TIME:
about 18 minutes·
CALORIES PER PORTION:
285 (1200 kilojoules)

1. Put the cubed lamb into
a shallow dish with the
peppercorns, salt, white
wine, orange rind,
cinnamon and sliced onion.
Cover and chill for 2 hours.
2. Drain the meat,
reserving the marinade,
and thread on to skewers.
3. Put the kebabs under a
preheated grill and grill for
4–5 minutes on each side.
4. Meanwhile make the
sauce. Fry the chopped
onion in the olive oil for 3
minutes. Add the strained
marinade and the saffron
and bubble briskly for 1
minute.
5. Blend the egg yolk with
the yogurt, orange juice
and cornflour; add to the
sauce and stir over a gentle
heat until lightly
thickened. Add a little
artificial sweetener if
necessary.
6. Serve the cooked kebabs
accompanied by the sauce.

JULY

Puddings

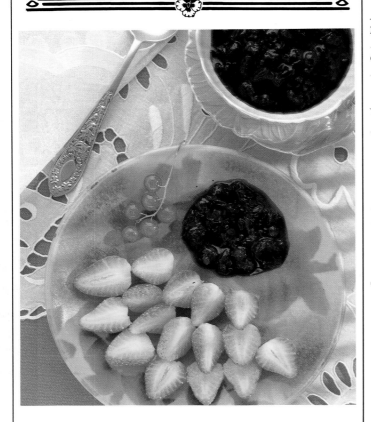

Stuffed Figs

*12 ripe fresh figs, preferably
  purple ones*
3 tablespoons ground almonds
100 g (4 oz) fresh raspberries
1 tablespoon honey
*4 vine leaves, soaked in warm
  water and dried, to serve*

PREPARATION TIME:
10–15 minutes
CALORIES PER PORTION:
130 (545 kilojoules)

1. Snip off any excess stalk
from each fig; make a criss-
cross cut down from the
stalk end and carefully
ease the cut open.
2. Mix the ground almonds
with the fresh raspberries
and honey.
3. Place a vine leaf, spread
out flat, on each serving
plate; arrange 3 figs on top
of each one, and fill with
the raspberry and almond
purée.

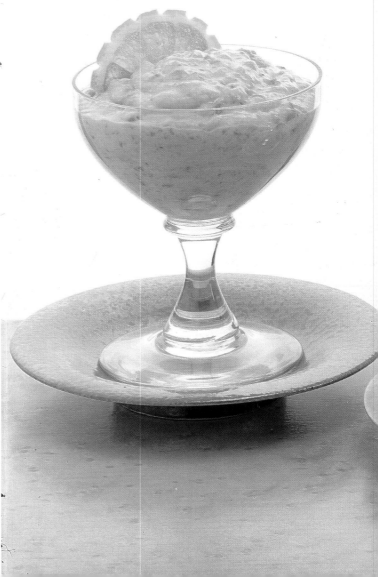

Strawberries with Blackcurrant Sauce

*225 g (8 oz) fresh
  blackcurrants, trimmed*
2 tablespoons honey
3 tablespoons red wine
*350 g (12 oz) ripe
  strawberries, hulled*
*small sprigs of fresh
  redcurrants, to decorate*

PREPARATION TIME:
25 minutes, plus cooling
COOKING TIME:
5 minutes
CALORIES PER PORTION:
75 (315 kilojoules)

1. Put the trimmed
blackcurrants into a pan
with the honey and red
wine; stir well then
simmer gently until the
natural fruit juices are
released (about 5
minutes).
2. Blend the lightly cooked
blackcurrants and their
liquid in the liquidizer
until fairly smooth – the
sauce should still have
some texture. Allow to
cool.
3. Arrange the halved
strawberries in small
decorative dishes and
spoon the blackcurrant
sauce near to them.
4. Decorate with clusters of
fresh redcurrants.

Greengage Fool

450 g (1 lb) ripe fresh
  greengages
juice of 1 orange
150 ml (¼ pint) skimmed
  milk
15 g (½ oz) cornflour
artificial sweetener, to taste
4 tablespoons plain
  unsweetened yogurt
halved orange slices, to
  garnish

PREPARATION TIME:
30 minutes, plus chilling
COOKING TIME:
10–15 minutes
CALORIES PER PORTION:
100 (420 kilojoules)

1. Put the greengages into a pan with the orange juice; cover the pan and simmer gently until the fruit is just tender. Remove all the stones and cool.

2. Blend 2 tablespoons of the milk with the cornflour; heat the remaining milk in a pan and then stir into the cornflour paste. Return to the saucepan and stir over a gentle heat until the sauce has thickened. Add a little sweetener to taste.
3. Cool the sauce and then mix it with the cooled greengages; stir in the yogurt.

4. Spoon into stemmed glass dishes and chill for 2 hours before serving.
5. Garnish each portion with a halved orange slice.

FAR LEFT Strawberries with blackcurrant sauce BELOW, FROM LEFT Greengage fool; Stuffed figs

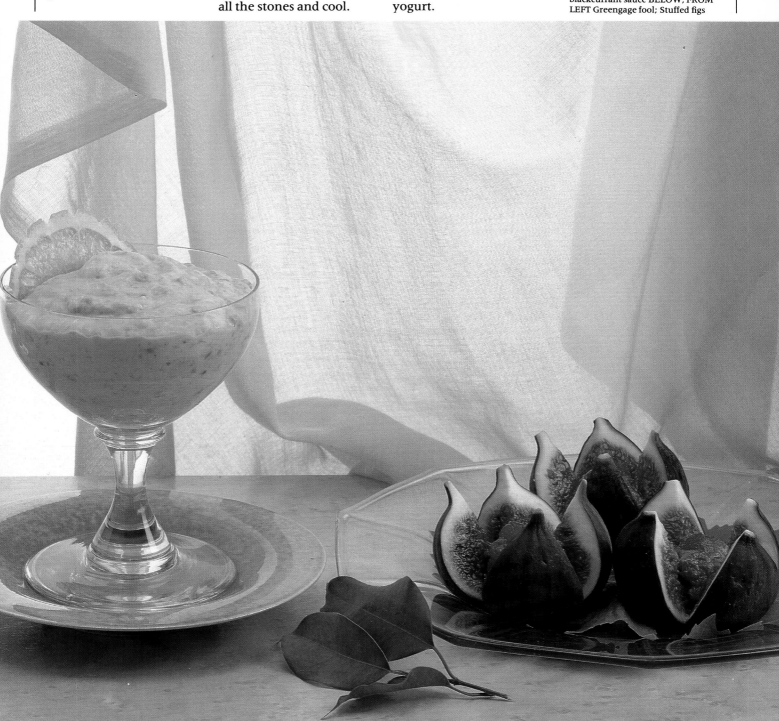

Dinner Party for Six

Estouffade de Boletus

450 g (1 lb) aubergines
salt
2 tablespoons sunflower oil
350 g (12 oz) onions, peeled
  and sliced
3 large garlic cloves, peeled
  and quartered
750 g (1½ lb) large flat
  mushrooms, preferably field
  mushrooms
2 × 400 g (14 oz) cans
  tomatoes
2½ tablespoons tomato purée
1 tablespoon red wine vinegar
1 teaspoon brown sugar
1 tablespoon soy sauce
freshly ground black pepper
2 bay leaves

PREPARATION TIME:
20 minutes, plus standing
COOKING TIME:
about 2 hours
CALORIES PER PORTION:
90 (380 kilojoules)

If you are fortunate enough to have the dried Italian mushrooms called *funghi porcini (Boletus edulis)* in your store cupboard, you will be able to make this dish as it was originally created. After soaking, these mushrooms have a unique meaty flavour, which is quite exquisite. Use field mushrooms instead and you will produce a dish very similar to the original and just as good.

1. Slice the aubergines into pieces approximately the size and shape of French fries (or use the chipper disc of a food processor). Transfer to a colander, sprinkle with salt, and set aside to drain.
2. Heat the oil in a large heavy-based pan and soften the onion and garlic.
3. Wipe the mushrooms and slice into strips about 1 cm (½ inch) wide.
4. Rinse the aubergine then squeeze to extract as much liquid as possible. Add the aubergines to the pan. Stir over a medium heat for about 1 minute, then add the mushrooms; stir and cover.
5. Push the tomatoes through a vegetable mill to remove the pips and add to the pan. Bring to a simmering point, cover and cook for 1 hour stirring occasionally.
6. Add the remaining ingredients. Stir thoroughly to dissolve the tomato purée, which will thicken the mixture, then continue to simmer uncovered for a further 45 minutes approximately. Taste and adjust the seasoning.
7. Remove from the heat, cover and leave to stand for up to 24 hours. Remove the bay leaves.
8. Serve cold, or very slightly warmed, with small wholemeal rolls.

Poussin de l'été

3 poussins, about 350 g
  (12 oz) each
salt
10 sprigs fresh basil
finely grated rind of 1 lemon
250 ml (8 fl oz) water
300 ml (10 fl oz) white wine
freshly ground black pepper

PREPARATION TIME:
8 minutes, plus cooling
COOKING TIME:
40 minutes
OVEN TEMPERATURE:
220°C, 425°F, Gas Mark 7
THEN:
180°C, 350°F, Gas Mark 4
CALORIES PER PORTION:
170 (710 kilojoules)

1. Wash the birds inside and out and rub with salt.
2. Strip the leaves off half the sprigs of basil and chop them roughly. Combine with the lemon rind.
3. Carefully lift the skin away from the breast of each poussin by pushing the fingers up through the neck cavity and easing them between the skin and the flesh, taking care not to tear the skin. Spread the basil and lemon rind over the breast under the skin.
4. Place the birds in an earthenware ovenproof dish and surround with the remaining sprigs of basil. Pour the water into the dish and pour the wine over. Sprinkle with salt and pepper.
5. Place, uncovered, in a preheated oven for 15 minutes, then cover, reduce the temperature and cook for a further 25 minutes. Remove and allow to cool completely. The liquids in the dish should have jellied.
6. Scrape off any fat which may have accumulated on top of the jelly. Serve one half poussin per head, with the jelly, mangetout and new potatoes.

Summer Pudding

225 g (8 oz) red and white
  currants, topped and tailed
100 g (4 oz) blackcurrants,
  topped and tailed
100 g (4 oz) raspberries, hulled
100 g (4 oz) loganberries,
  hulled
100 g (4 oz) strawberries,
  hulled
100 g (4 oz) cherries,
  blueberries or cultivated
  blackberries
1 tablespoon honey
1 sachet gelatine (optional)
8 × 1 cm (½ inch) thick slices
  brown bread, crusts removed
  (see below)

PREPARATION TIME:
30 minutes, plus chilling
COOKING TIME:
3 minutes
CALORIES PER PORTION:
190 (790 kilojoules)

This classic English pudding is made with a selection of summer soft fruits which you can vary as you choose. The addition of gelatine makes the serving of the pudding much easier. Use one of the softer, lighter types of brown bread for this recipe.

1. Place all the fruit in a large saucepan (it must not be aluminium or cast iron) with the honey and cook very gently for 2–3 minutes, just long enough to soften the fruit and cause the juices to run a little.
2. Sprinkle the gelatine over and stir it in very carefully, trying not to crush the fruit.
3. Line a lightly greased 1.2 litre (2 pint) pudding basin with three-quarters of the bread, trimming the slices to fit, making certain that all the surfaces are completely covered and

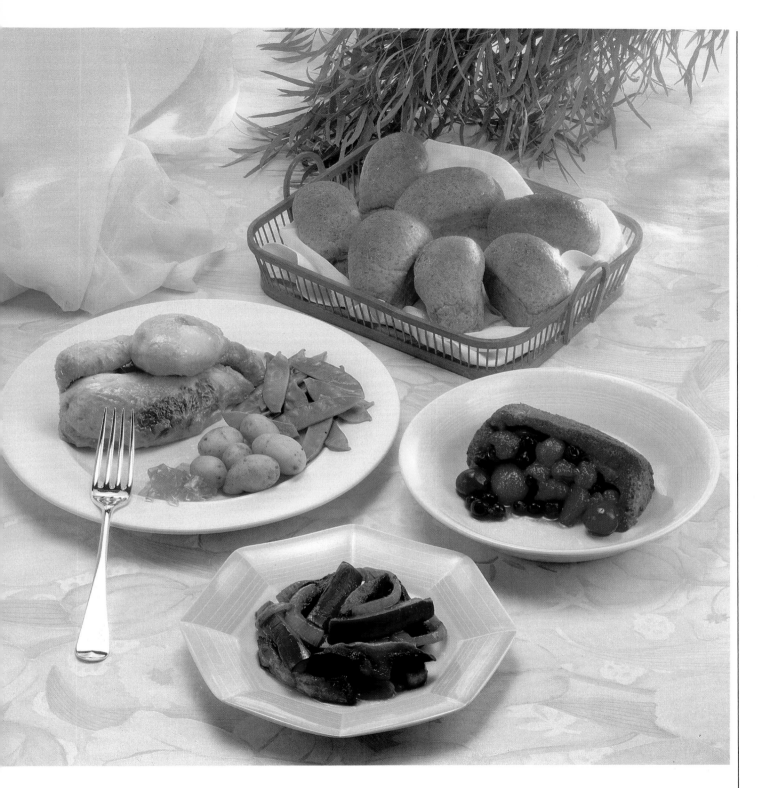

the bottom has an extra thick layer.

4. Spoon in all the fruit, reserving 2 tablespoons of the juice in case the bread is not completely coloured by the fruit when the pudding is turned out. Cover with the remaining bread. Lay a plate or saucepan lid that will fit inside the rim of the bowl on top and place a 1 kg (2 lb) weight on top. Chill for 10–12 hours.

5. Turn out and cut into wedges to serve.

CLOCKWISE FROM BOTTOM
Estouffade de boletus; Poussin de l'été; Summer pudding

AUGUST

Barbecue for Ten

Let your guests cook their own kebabs which you have prepared; this way you are not still slaving over the hot coals while everyone is enjoying their meal. Remember to light the barbecue well ahead of time.

Chick Pea Salad

2 onions, peeled and finely chopped
1 teaspoon fresh thyme
1 tablespoon olive oil
2 medium red peppers, cored, seeded and finely chopped
3 × 400 g (14 oz) cans chick peas, drained and rinsed
50 g (2 oz) seedless raisins
salt
freshly ground black pepper
2–3 tablespoons vinegar

PREPARATION TIME:
15 minutes, plus chilling overnight
COOKING TIME:
10 minutes
CALORIES PER PORTION:
230 (960 kilojoules)

---

1. Fry the onions with the thyme in the oil until pale golden.
2. Add the red peppers and cook for 5 minutes, then add the chick peas and raisins and cook for a further 4–5 minutes, stirring gently.
3. Add salt and pepper then transfer to a serving dish. Pour over the vinegar while still hot. Allow to cool uncovered.
4. When cold, cover and refrigerate for 24 hours.
5. Bring the salad to room temperature to serve.

Monkfish Kebabs

2 kg (4½ lb) monkfish, cut into 4 cm (1½ inch) cubes
1 teaspoon salt
4 tablespoons white wine
2 tablespoons lemon juice
1 sprig fresh rosemary, needles removed and chopped
1 garlic clove, peeled and crushed
3 lemons, cut into small chunks
4 green peppers, seeded and cut into small rectangles
5 pitta breads, halved and warmed, to serve (optional)

PREPARATION TIME:
10 minutes, plus marinating
COOKING TIME:
10 minutes
CALORIES PER PORTION:
200 (825 kilojoules)

---

1. Sprinkle the monkfish with salt and pour over the wine and lemon juice. Stir in the rosemary and garlic, cover and marinate for 1 hour.
2. Thread cubes of fish, chunks of lemon and pepper pieces alternately on to 10 skewers. Lay the skewers on a dish, sprinkle some of the marinade over and cover with foil.
3. When the charcoal is ready for cooking, place the skewers on the barbecue rack and cook for 10 minutes, turning frequently.
4. Serve the kebabs, in pockets of warm pitta bread if liked.

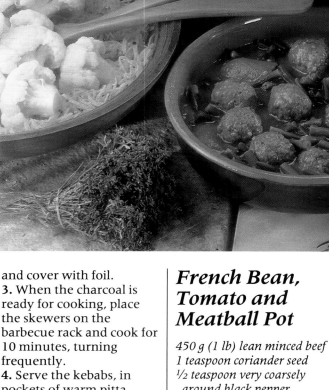

French Bean, Tomato and Meatball Pot

450 g (1 lb) lean minced beef
1 teaspoon coriander seed
½ teaspoon very coarsely ground black pepper
½ teaspoon cumin seed
½ teaspoon salt
1 tablespoon red wine vinegar
oil
3 × 400g (14 oz) cans tomatoes
1 bay leaf
1 dried chilli
1 kg (2 lb) French beans, chopped into 2 cm (¾ inch) lengths
1 tablespoon red wine

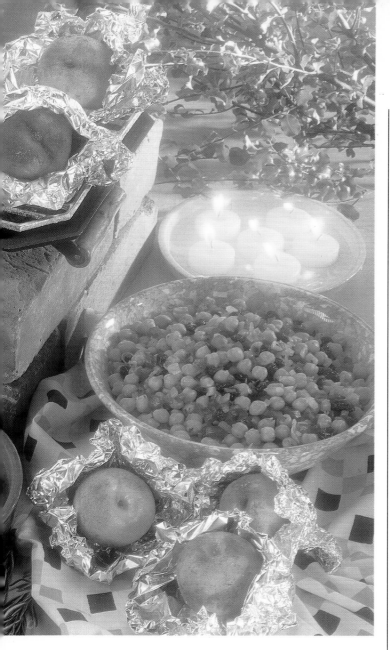

Carrot and Cauliflower Mint Salad

2 large bunches mint, washed
2 medium cauliflowers, broken into florets
½ teaspoon caster sugar
225 g (8 oz) carrots, coarsely grated
2 teaspoons black mustard seed
1 tablespoon olive oil
2 tablespoons lemon juice
salt
pepper

PREPARATION TIME:
15 minutes, plus chilling
COOKING TIME:
8–10 minutes
CALORIES PER PORTION:
20 (88 kilojoules)

1. Put the mint on a steamer, bed in the cauliflower and steam it for 8 minutes or so until tender but still crisp. Allow it to cool still covered in the mint.
2. Mix the sugar into the carrots.
3. Put the mustard seed in a pan with the olive oil and fry it until it has stopped popping, then mix it into the carrot. Discard the mint and combine the carrots and cauliflower together in a salad bowl.
4. Sprinkle the lemon juice over, season with salt and pepper and chill until ready to serve.

Hot Spiced Peaches

1 tablespoon caster sugar
1 teaspoon ground cinnamon
½ teaspoon ground allspice
2 pinches of ground cloves
1 teaspoon finely grated lemon rind
1 teaspoon finely grated orange rind
½ teaspoon grated nutmeg
½ teaspoon ground ginger
10 peaches, skinned

PREPARATION TIME:
20 minutes
COOKING TIME:
10–15 minutes
CALORIES PER PORTION:
40 (170 kilojoules)

1. Cut 10 pieces of foil into squares large enough completely to encase the peaches.
2. Mix all the ingredients except the peaches together in a bowl. Place a portion of mixture on each square of foil.
3. Roll each peach in the spiced sugar and seal them completely by folding up the foil and twisting the corners together. Cook on the barbecue for about 10–15 minutes, depending on how hot the barbecue coals are.
4. Serve in the foil.

PREPARATION TIME:
30 minutes
COOKING TIME:
20–30 minutes
CALORIES PER PORTION:
135 (560 kilojoules)

To be able to cook this dish out of doors you need a flameproof earthenware or terracotta casserole that you don't mind blackening a little. If more practical, the pot can be cooked in an oven preheated to 200°C, 400°F, Gas Mark 6 for 40 minutes, having first sealed the meatballs on top of the stove.

1. Place the minced beef in a bowl and add the coriander, black pepper, cumin seed, salt and vinegar. Oil your hands and knead the mixture for a minute before forming walnut-sized balls.
2. Carefully imbed the casserole in the coals. Allow to heat up then add 2 teaspoons oil. Put in the meat, a few balls at a time, stirring to seal them. Add the tomatoes, bay leaf and chilli.
3. Stir from time to time and boil for about 5 minutes, then add the French beans and red wine. Cook uncovered for 15–25 minutes, until the beans are just tender.

CLOCKWISE FROM TOP LEFT
Monkfish kebabs; Hot spiced peaches; Chick pea salad; French bean, tomato and meatball pot; Carrot and cauliflower mint salad

AUGUST

Hors d'oeuvres and Light Meals

Smoked Chicken with Peach Purée

3 ripe peaches
3 tablespoons dry Vermouth
1 teaspoon French mustard
1 teaspoon chopped fresh
* tarragon*
salt
freshly ground black pepper
12 thin slices smoked chicken,
* about 175–225 g (6–8 oz) in*
* total weight*
To garnish:
thin slices of fresh peach
small sprigs of fresh tarragon

PREPARATION TIME:
25 minutes, plus chilling
CALORIES PER PORTION:
140 (590 kilojoules)

1. Nick the stalk end of each peach; plunge into a bowl of boiling water for 45 seconds, then slide off the skins, remove the stones and chop the flesh.
2. Blend the peach flesh in the liquidizer with the Vermouth, mustard, chopped tarragon, and a little salt and pepper.
3. Cover the sauce and chill for 1 hour. (Do not chill any longer to avoid discoloration.)
4. Spoon a little of the sauce on to each plate; lay 4 slices of chicken in a fan shape close by.
5. Garnish with slices of peach and sprigs of tarragon.

Chilled Tomato and Basil Soup

1 kg (2 lb) ripe tomatoes,
* skinned, seeded and chopped*
1 large garlic clove, peeled
* and finely chopped*
1 tablespoon chopped fresh
* basil*
450 ml (¾ pint) chicken stock
juice of 1 large orange
2 anchovy fillets, chopped
salt
freshly ground black pepper
Pesto croûtes:
4 thin slices wholemeal bread
2 teaspoons Pesto sauce

PREPARATION TIME:
15–20 minutes, plus chilling
COOKING TIME:
6–7 minutes
CALORIES PER PORTION:
125 (525 kilojoules)

1. Put the tomatoes into a pan with the garlic, basil, stock, orange juice, anchovy fillets and salt and pepper to taste.
2. Bring to the boil and simmer for 3–4 minutes.
3. Cool slightly and then liquidize until smooth. Chill for at least 4 hours.
4. To make the Pesto croûtes, spread each slice of wholemeal bread with a thin layer of Pesto sauce; place under a preheated grill until a light golden brown. Cut into fingers.
5. Ladle the soup into bowls and serve with the Pesto croûtes.

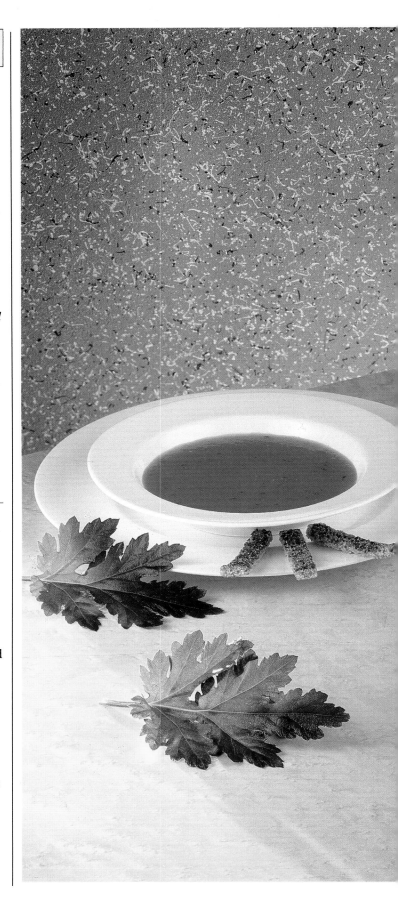

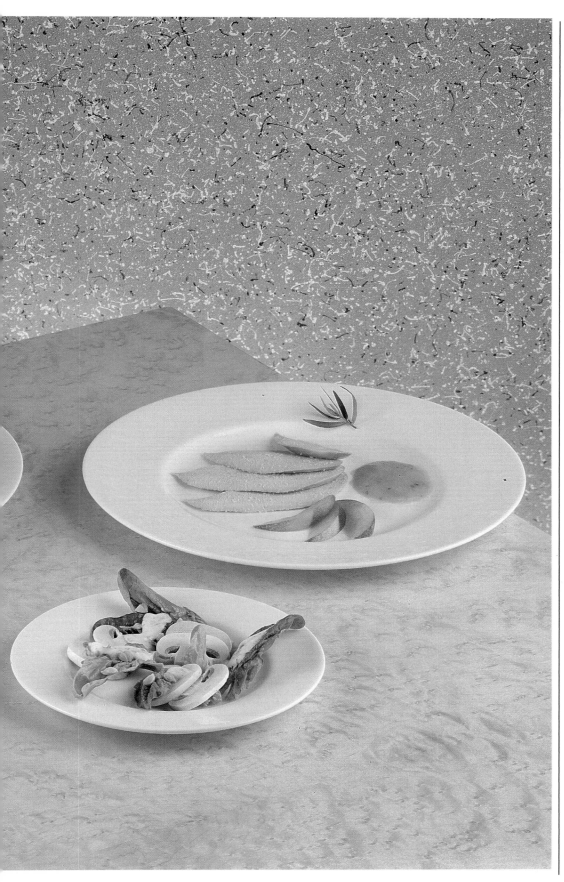

Spinach, Mushroom and Hazelnut Salad

2 tablespoons olive oil
2 tablespoons white wine
  vinegar
1 garlic clove, peeled and
  chopped
2 tablespoons roughly
  chopped parsley
3 tablespoons plain
  unsweetened yogurt
salt
freshly ground black pepper
175 g (6 oz) young fresh
  spinach leaves, washed and
  shaken
100 g (4 oz) button
  mushrooms, thinly sliced
50 g (2 oz) hazelnuts, coarsely
  chopped

PREPARATION TIME:
15 minutes
CALORIES PER PORTION:
140 (590 kilojoules)

1. To make the dressing,
put the olive oil, wine
vinegar, garlic, parsley,
yogurt, and salt and pepper
to taste into a liquidizer;
blend until smooth.
2. Tear the spinach leaves
into pieces and divide
among 4 individual salad
plates.
3. Scatter the mushrooms
and hazelnuts over the
spinach. Spoon the
prepared dressing over
each serving, and toss
lightly.

FROM THE LEFT Chilled tomato and
basil soup; Spinach, mushroom and
hazelnut salad; Smoked chicken with
peach purée

AUGUST

Main Courses

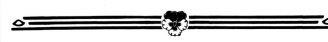

Lettuce Parcels with Avocado and Pimento Sauce

1 ripe avocado pear
1 garlic clove, peeled and chopped
1 canned red pimento, drained and roughly chopped
1 tablespoon lemon juice
finely grated rind of ½ lemon
150 ml (¼ pint) chicken stock
salt
freshly ground black pepper
8 tablespoons cooked brown rice
3 spring onions, finely chopped
3 hard-boiled eggs, shelled and finely chopped
175 g (6 oz) cottage cheese, sieved
1 tablespoon chopped fresh tarragon
2 tablespoons low calorie mayonnaise
16 good-shaped leaves from a round lettuce
To garnish:
12 mangetout, blanched
1 small red pepper, cored, seeded and cut into matchstick strips

PREPARATION TIME:
45 minutes, plus chilling
CALORIES PER PORTION:
435 (1820 kilojoules)

1. Peel, halve and stone the avocado; chop the flesh and put into the liquidizer with the garlic, chopped pimento, lemon juice and rind, chicken stock and salt and pepper to taste; blend until smooth. Cover and chill for 2 hours.
2. Mix the cooked rice with the spring onions, hard-boiled egg, cottage cheese, tarragon, mayonnaise and salt and pepper to taste.
3. Trim the excess stalk from the lettuce leaves. (This will make them more pliable.)
4. Cup one lettuce leaf in your hand; place ⅛ of the rice mixture in the centre, and fold the lettuce over and around it. Wrap another lettuce leaf over the top, and place 'seam-side' down in a shallow serving dish, or a platter with a rim.
5. Repeat with the remaining lettuce leaves and rice filling, so that you have 8 parcels in all.
6. Spoon the prepared sauce over the lettuce parcels – if the sauce seems too thick, thin it down with extra chicken stock. Chill for 1 hour.
7. Garnish with mangetout and strips of red pepper.

Sole Tonnato

1 × 200 g (7 oz) can tuna fish in brine
1 tablespoon capers
4 anchovy fillets, chopped
grated rind and juice of ½ lemon
salt
freshly ground black pepper
200 ml (⅓ pint) low calorie mayonnaise
25 g (1 oz) butter
8 small sole fillets, about 65 g (2½ oz) each
75 ml (⅛ pint) white wine
chicken stock
To garnish:
1 tablespoon capers
4 anchovy fillets
thin lemon slices

PREPARATION TIME:
10–15 minutes, plus chilling
COOKING TIME:
5 minutes, plus chilling
CALORIES PER PORTION:
390 (1630 kilojoules)

1. Drain the tuna fish. Put it into a liquidizer with the capers, chopped anchovy fillets, lemon rind and juice, salt and pepper to taste and the mayonnaise; blend until smooth. Cover and keep chilled.
2. Heat the butter in a large shallow frying pan; add the sole fillets and fry gently for 1 minute. Turn the fillets over carefully and fry for a further minute. Add the white wine, salt and pepper to taste and sufficient stock to half cover. Allow to bubble gently for 2–3 minutes.
3. Remove the fish fillets with a slice and place on a serving platter.
4. Add sufficient of the fish cooking liquid to the prepared tonnato sauce to give a thickish coating consistency. Spoon over the fish while it is still warm. Chill for 1 hour.
5. Garnish with capers, anchovy fillets and lemon.

Stir-Fried Beef with Peppers

1 tablespoon olive oil
1 medium onion, peeled and thinly sliced
1 large garlic clove, peeled and cut into thin strips
450 g (1 lb) fillet steak, cut into thin strips
1 red pepper, seeded and cut into matchstick strips
1 green pepper, seeded and cut into matchstick strips
1 tablespoon soy sauce
2 tablespoons dry sherry
salt
freshly ground black pepper
1 tablespoon chopped fresh rosemary

PREPARATION TIME:
5 minutes
COOKING TIME:
10–12 minutes
CALORIES PER PORTION:
90 (380 kilojoules)

1. Heat the olive oil in a wok or deep frying pan and stir-fry the onion and garlic for 2 minutes.
2. Add the strips of beef and stir-fry briskly until evenly browned on all sides and almost tender.
3. Add the strips of red and green pepper and stir-fry for a further 2 minutes.
4. Add the soy sauce, sherry, salt and pepper to taste and the rosemary, and stir-fry for a further 1–2 minutes.
5. Serve piping hot with brown rice.

CLOCKWISE FROM TOP Sole tonnato; Lettuce parcels with avocado and pimento sauce; Stir-fried beef with peppers

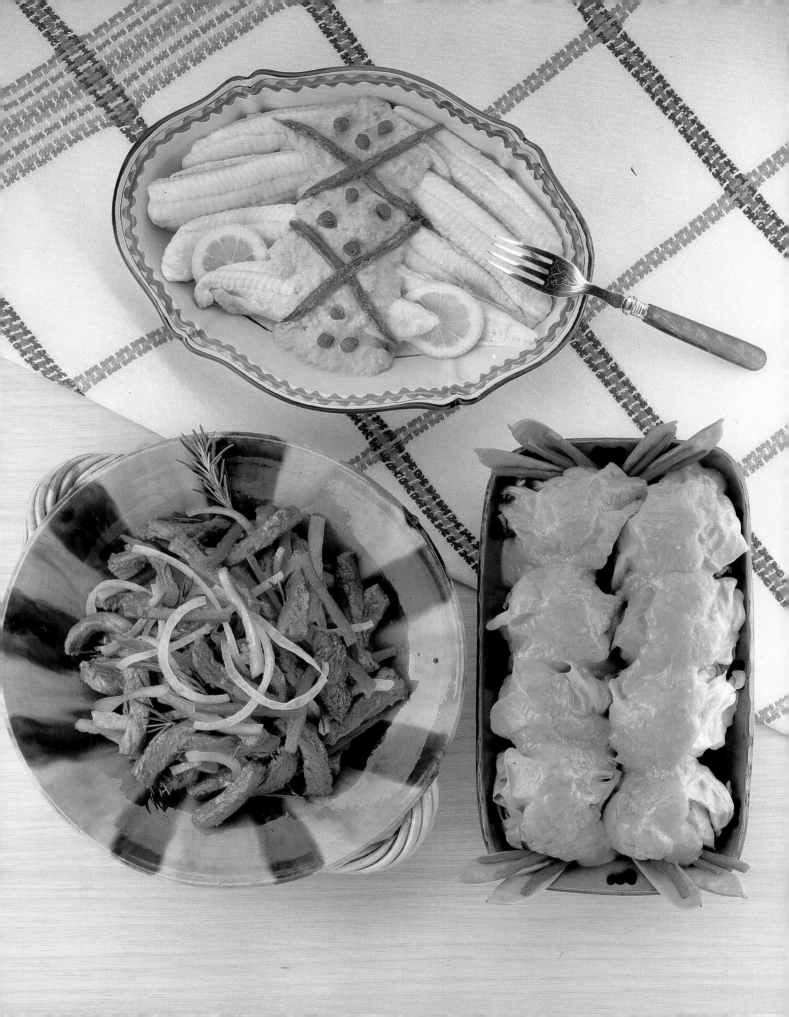

AUGUST

Puddings

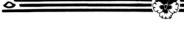

Pears with Fresh Raspberry Sauce

4 large firm pears
300 ml (½ pint) orange juice
bay leaf
small piece of cinnamon stick
1 tablespoon clear honey
225 g (8 oz) fresh raspberries

PREPARATION TIME:
about 20 minutes, plus cooling
COOKING TIME:
10 minutes
CALORIES PER PORTION:
120 (505 kilojoules)

1. Peel, halve and core the pears. Place them in a saucepan with the orange juice, bay leaf, cinnamon stick and honey. Cover the pan and simmer gently for 10 minutes.
2. Turn the pear halves over in their cooking liquid; cover the pan and leave them to cool in their liquid.
3. Blend the raspberries in the liquidizer until smooth; add sufficient of the pear cooking liquid to give a thin coating consistency.
4. Arrange the drained pear halves in a shallow serving dish and trickle over the prepared sauce.

Variation:
Spoon the raspberry sauce on to individual serving plates; trickle a little plain unsweetened yogurt on top, and arrange the pear halves carefully on top. Calories per portion: 135 (570 kilojoules).

Blushing Plums

200 ml (⅓ pint) red wine
1 tablespoon clear honey
juice of 1 orange
100 g (4 oz) redcurrants, trimmed
12 really ripe plums, halved and stoned
sprigs of fresh lemon verbena or fresh plum leaves, to decorate

PREPARATION TIME:
15–20 minutes
COOKING TIME:
5 minutes
CALORIES PER PORTION:
110 (460 kilojoules)

1. Put the red wine, honey, orange juice and redcurrants into a pan; simmer for 5 minutes. Blend in the liquidizer until smooth then strain.
2. Arrange the plum halves in a shallow dish, and decorate the rim with lemon verbena or plum leaves. Spoon over the prepared redcurrant sauce.

Blackcurrant Cream

350 g (12 oz) fresh blackcurrants, trimmed
2 tablespoons clear honey
1 tablespoon brandy
2 egg yolks
1 teaspoon powdered gelatine
1 tablespoon water
200 ml (⅓ pint) plain unsweetened yogurt
borage flowers or small clusters of fresh blackcurrants, to decorate

PREPARATION TIME:
20 minutes, plus chilling
COOKING TIME:
8 minutes
CALORIES PER PORTION:
125 (525 kilojoules)

1. Put the blackcurrants into a pan with the honey and brandy; simmer gently for 8 minutes until the fruit is soft. Allow to cool.
2. Blend the cooked blackcurrants in the liquidizer until smooth; blend in the egg yolks.
3. Dissolve the gelatine in the water; beat into the blackcurrant mixture, together with the yogurt.
4. Spoon into dishes or stemmed glasses and chill for 1–2 hours until set.
5. Decorate each dessert with borage flowers or a cluster of fresh blackcurrants.

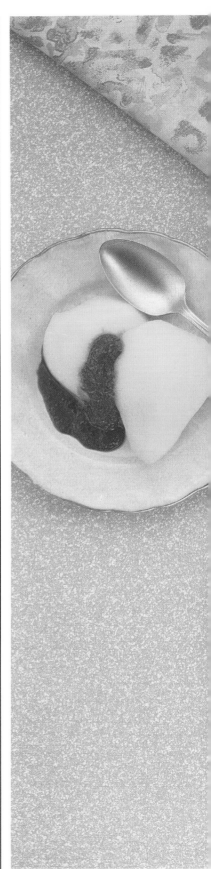

CLOCKWISE FROM TOP Blushing plums; Blackcurrant cream; Pears with fresh raspberry sauce

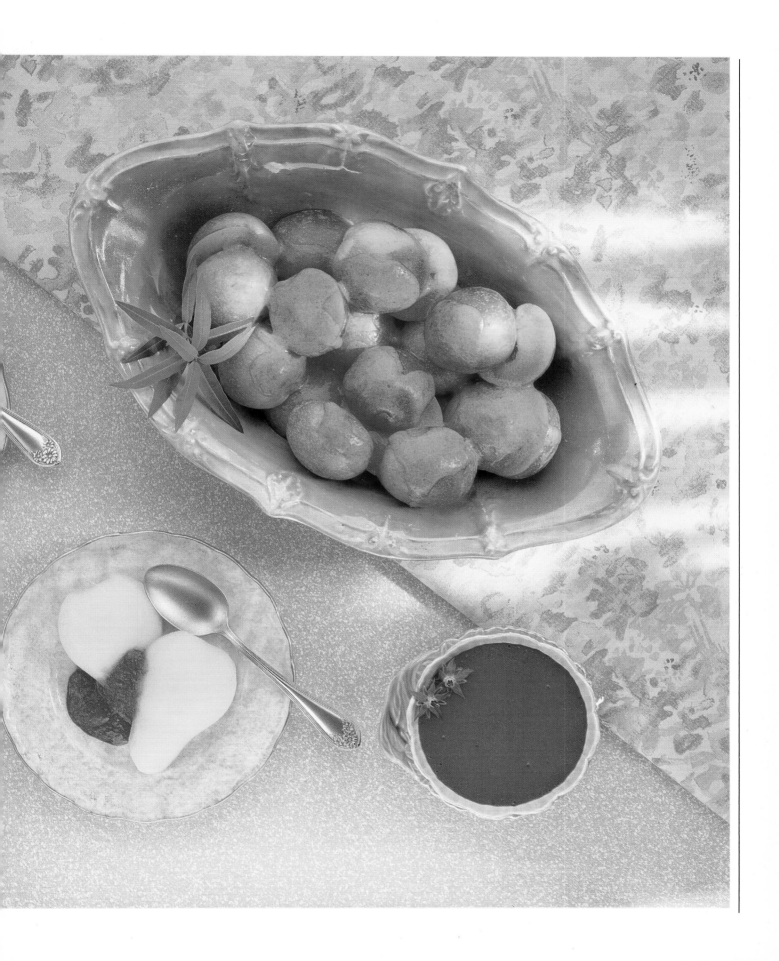

AUGUST

Dinner Party for Six

Basil and Potato Soup

15 g (½ oz) butter
750 g (1½ lb) floury potatoes, peeled and grated
6 garlic cloves, peeled
50 g (2 oz) fresh basil, chopped
600 ml (1 pint) chicken stock
600 ml (1 pint) dry white wine
1 teaspoon lemon juice
salt
freshly ground black pepper
15 g (½ oz) pine nuts, ground

PREPARATION TIME:
10 minutes, plus chilling
COOKING TIME:
20 minutes
CALORIES PER PORTION:
160 (670 kilojoules)

1. Heat the butter in a large heavy-based saucepan and add the potatoes, garlic and half the basil. Stir over a gentle heat for a couple of minutes, then add the stock and wine.
2. Bring to the boil and cook uncovered for 15 minutes, until all the

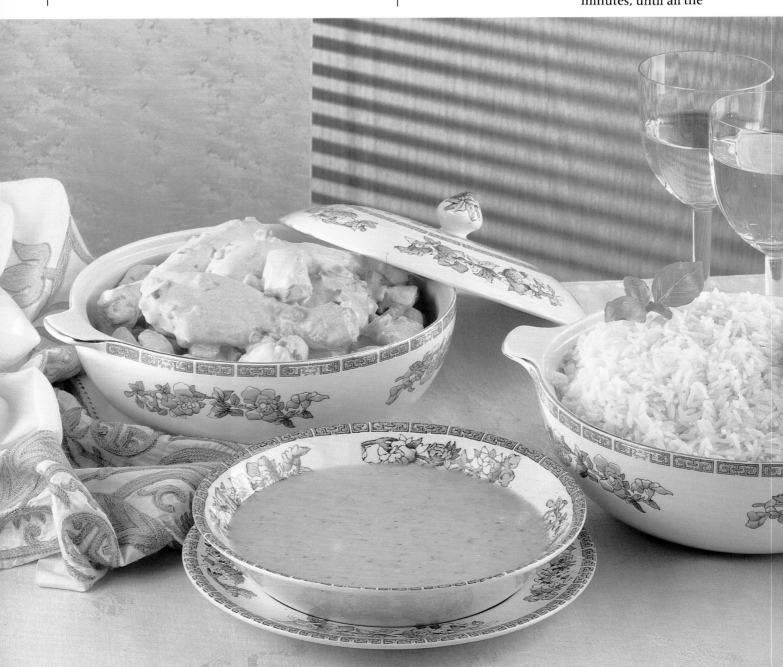

potatoes are quite soft.
3. Liquidize the soup, adding the remaining basil at the same time.
4. Taste and add lemon juice, salt and pepper to taste, remembering that if the soup is to be served chilled the seasoning will need to be a little more pronounced.
5. Mix the ground pine nuts with 2 tablespoons of the soup and stir into the soup. Chill thoroughly.

BELOW, FROM LEFT Spiced chicken; Basil and potato soup

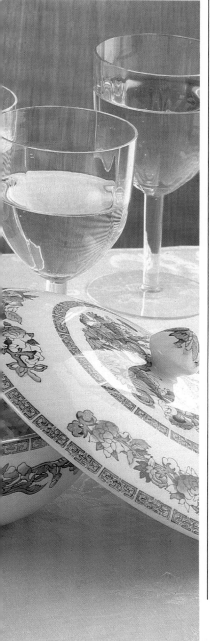

Spiced Chicken

1 teaspoon coarsely ground cinnamon
6 chicken drumsticks, skinned
3 boned and skinned chicken breasts, about 150 g (5 oz) each, cut into cubes
300 ml (½ pint) plain unsweetened yogurt
1 tablespoon oil
2 large onions, chopped
2 fresh green chillis, seeded and chopped
1 teaspoon cumin seed
1 garlic clove, peeled and chopped
1 tablespoon sweet paprika
2 tablespoons chicken stock
½ teaspoon finely grated lemon rind
1 red pepper, cored and chopped
1 tablespoon cornflour
salt
freshly ground black pepper

PREPARATION TIME:
10 minutes, plus marinating
COOKING TIME:
about 1¼ hours
CALORIES PER PORTION:
200 (825 kilojoules)

1. Rub the cinnamon into the chicken meat, combine with the yogurt and marinate for about 30 minutes.
2. Heat the oil in a casserole and lightly fry the onions, chillis, cumin and garlic. Stir in the paprika.
3. Strain the chicken meat, reserving the yogurt.
4. Add the chicken to the casserole, stir well to coat and then add the stock, lemon rind, red pepper and half of the reserved yogurt. Cover and simmer slowly for about 1 hour.
5. A few minutes before serving, combine the cornflour with the remaining yogurt and stir it into the casserole, bring to the boil and simmer for 1–2 minutes. Taste and add salt and pepper.
6. Serve with rice.

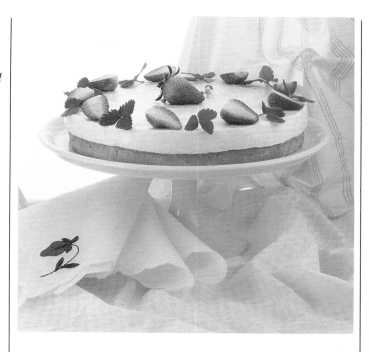

Strawberry Cheesecake

4 eggs (size 1), separated
50 g (2 oz) sugar
25 g (1 oz) plain flour, sifted
2 tablespoons very hot water
1 tablespoon lemon juice
1 sachet powdered gelatine
900 ml (1½ pints) very low fat soft cheese
½ teaspoon finely grated lemon rind
fresh strawberries (with leaves if available), to decorate

PREPARATION TIME:
45 minutes, plus chilling overnight
COOKING TIME:
about 18 minutes
OVEN TEMPERATURE:
180°C, 350°F, Gas Mark 4
CALORIES PER PORTION:
190 (790 kilojoules)

1. Line a 23 cm (9 inch) springform tin with non-stick silicone paper.
2. Cream the yolks of 2 eggs with half the sugar until very light and creamy.
3. Whip 2 egg whites until stiff and, with the flour, fold into the creamed yolks. Spread the mixture

ABOVE Strawberry cheesecake

evenly in the cake tin and bake in a preheated oven for 18 minutes until really firm, almost crisp.
4. Leave to cool in the tin, then remove. Re-line the tin with fresh paper. Drop the sponge back in the tin.
5. Combine the water, lemon juice and gelatine in a small bowl. Stand in a pan of hot water and stir until dissolved.
6. Put the cheese in a bowl and fold in the lemon rind.
7. Whisk the remaining 2 egg yolks with half the remaining sugar until very creamy. Slowly pour in the cooled gelatine mixture while still whisking. Combine with the cheese.
8. Whip the egg whites until firm, then add the remaining sugar and continue whipping until stiff. Fold into the mixture. Carefully and lightly turn the mixture into the cake tin, spreading it over the base. Chill overnight.
9. Carefully remove the sides of the tin and decorate with the fresh strawberries.

Side Salads

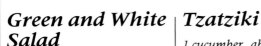

Green and White Salad

400 g (14 oz) young turnips,
no more than 5 cm (2 inches)
across, peeled
50 g (2 oz) roughly chopped
fresh parsley
4 tablespoons cultured
buttermilk or plain
unsweetened yogurt
1 tablespoon lemon juice
1 tablespoon chopped fresh
chives
pinch of salt (optional)
freshly ground black pepper
paprika, for dusting
(optional)

PREPARATION TIME:
8 minutes
CALORIES PER SERVING:
about 40 (175 kilojoules)

Small young turnips are
deliciously sweet.

1. Cut the turnips into
paper-thin slices directly
into a serving bowl, using a
mandoline if possible.
2. Stir in all the remaining
ingredients except the
paprika.
3. Dust lightly with
paprika, if liked, just before
serving.

Tzatziki

1 cucumber, about 450 g
(1 lb), peeled
300 ml (½ pint) thick plain
unsweetened yogurt
2 tablespoons lemon juice
2 tablespoons chopped fresh
spring onions or chives
2 tablespoons chopped fresh
parsley
1 tablespoon chopped fresh
mint
1–2 garlic cloves, peeled and
crushed, or 1 shallot, peeled
and finely chopped
freshly ground black pepper
large pinch of salt
To serve:
100 g (4 oz) wholemeal pitta
bread, warmed and cut into
fingers

PREPARATION TIME:
10 minutes
CALORIES PER SERVING:
about 117 (490 kilojoules)

A salad that is frequently
served as a first course in
Greece. The cucumber can
be successfully exchanged
for coarsely grated carrot,
fennel, celery mixed with
apple, Cos lettuce or
mushrooms.

1. Chop the cucumber
finely.
2. Mix all the other
ingredients together and
combine with the
cucumber in a serving
bowl.
3. Serve with the pitta
bread fingers.

Tomatoes with Basil

450 g (1 lb) tomatoes, thickly
sliced
25 g (1 oz) pine nuts or
almond flakes
about 5 large fresh basil
leaves
1 tablespoon walnut oil or
virgin (first pressing) olive oil
1–2 tablespoons lemon juice,
to taste
1 clove garlic, peeled and
crushed (optional)
150 ml (¼ pint) cultured
buttermilk, smetana or
unsweetened low fat yogurt
freshly ground black pepper
sea salt
tiny fresh basil leaves, to
garnish

PREPARATION TIME:
10 minutes
CALORIES PER SERVING:
about 110 (460 kilojoules)

Fresh basil's wonderful
flavour is lost in drying. If
unavailable use fresh dill
or tarragon leaves instead.
Here, basil is combined
with its traditional Italian
partners of walnut or olive
oil, garlic and pine nuts.

1. Arrange the tomatoes on
a flat serving dish.
2. Place the pine nuts or
almonds in an ungreased
heavy-based pan and stir
over a low heat for 2–3
minutes until lightly
browned. Sprinkle over
the tomato slices.
3. In a liquidizer, blend the
basil, oil, lemon juice and
garlic together, adding the
lemon juice little by little,
to taste. Transfer to a jug.
4. Stir the buttermilk,
smetana or yogurt into the
mixture. Add pepper and
salt to taste.
5. To serve, sprinkle the
tiny basil leaves over the
tomato slices and hand the
sauce separately.

Broad Bean Salad

450 g (1 lb) fresh or frozen
broad beans, shelled weight
1–2 teaspoons chopped fresh
summer savory, dill or
tarragon
4 spring onions, trimmed and
finely chopped
1 tablespoon horseradish
sauce
150 ml (¼ pint) plain
unsweetened yogurt
pinch of salt
pinch of pepper
sprig of fresh summer savory,
dill or tarragon, to garnish

PREPARATION TIME:
15 minutes
CALORIES PER SERVING:
about 86 (358 kilojoules)

When broad beans are
very young, you can slice
and cook the whole pod. If
you can obtain fresh grated
horseradish, use ½–1
teaspoon instead of
horseradish sauce.

1. If using fresh beans,
plunge them into 1 cm
(½ inch) boiling water in a
saucepan. Bring back to
the boil, cover and simmer
for 10–12 minutes. If using
frozen beans, cook according to the instructions on
the packet. Drain.
2. Mix all the other ingredients together in a serving
dish.
3. Toss the warm beans in
the dressing. Taste, and
add a little more horse-
radish or salt if necessary.
Serve immediately,
garnished with a sprig of
summer savory, dill or
tarragon.

FROM THE TOP Broad bean salad;
Tomatoes with basil; Green and white
salad; Tzatziki

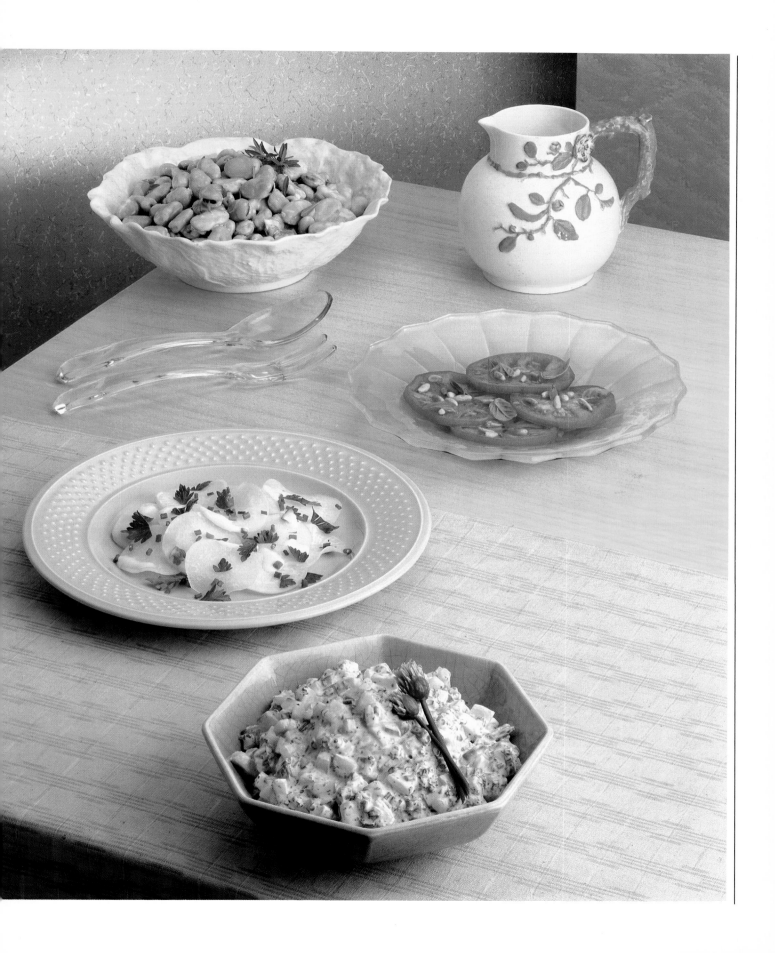

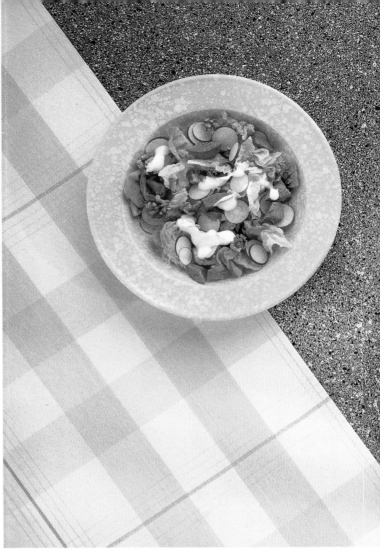

Main Course Salads

Californian Salad

1 kg (2 lb) assorted fruit
(choose from apricots,
cherries, grapefruit, kiwi
fruit, melon, nectarines,
peaches, raspberries and
strawberries)
50 g (2 oz) chopped nuts
450 g (1 lb) cottage cheese
2 bananas
1 tablespoon lemon juice

PREPARATION TIME:
15 minutes
CALORIES PER SERVING:
about 325 (1350 kilojoules)

1. Prepare all the fruit
(except the bananas),
peeling, slicing, stoning
and hulling as necessary.
2. Combine all the
prepared fruit in a large
bowl.
3. Toast the nuts under a
preheated medium grill for
2 minutes until lightly
browned.
4. Peel the bananas, cut
into long diagonal slices
and immediately toss in
the lemon juice to prevent
discoloration. Add the
banana slices to the other
fruit.
5. Spoon the cottage
cheese into the centre of
the fruit in the bowl and
sprinkle the chopped nuts
over it. Serve immediately.

Chicker Liver and Walnut Salad

5 teaspoons olive or walnut oil
450 g (1 lb) chicken livers
25 g (1 oz) walnut pieces
1 clove garlic, peeled and
crushed (optional)
2 teaspoons wine vinegar
3 tablespoons plain
unsweetened yogurt
pinch of salt
pinch of black pepper
½ lettuce, washed and torn
into pieces
50 g (2 oz) radishes, trimmed
and sliced very thinly
4 spring onions, trimmed and
finely chopped

PREPARATION TIME:
15 minutes
COOKING TIME:
10 minutes
CALORIES PER SERVING:
about 270 (1130 kilojoules)

Walnut oil is extravagant
but well worth using in
this unusual warm salad.

1. Brush a thick saucepan
with 1 teaspoon of the oil,
and heat gently. With
kitchen scissors, snip the
chicken livers into
quarters, directly into the
pan, cutting off and
discarding any green parts.
Stir over a medium heat
for 4 minutes.
2. Add the walnut pieces,
turn the heat down as far
as possible, cover tightly
and simmer for a further 5

minutes. The livers should
be just cooked and still
slightly pink inside.
3. Meanwhile, blend the
remaining oil with the
garlic (if using), vinegar,
yogurt, salt and pepper in a
jug.
4. Place the lettuce,
radishes and spring onions
in a bowl and toss well.
5. Divide the vegetable
mixture between 4 shallow
bowls or dinner plates.
Spoon the liver quarters
with the walnuts and pan
juices over the vegetables
and serve, accompanied by
the dressing.

CLOCKWISE FROM TOP LEFT
Chicken liver and walnut salad;
Ceviche; Californian salad; Hummus
with pitta bread and vegetable strips

Ceviche

500 g (1 lb 2 oz) white fish,
boned and cut into bite-size
chunks
175 ml (6 fl oz) combined lime
and lemon juice
2 onions, peeled and finely
sliced
1 chilli pepper, finely sliced
(or to taste)
50 g (2 oz) fresh coconut
slivers (optional)
4 tablespoons plain
unsweetened yogurt or
smetana
2 tablespoons chopped fresh
chives
1 teaspoon finely grated fresh
ginger
pinch of salt
½ crisp lettuce, washed
To serve:
1 lime, cut into 8 wedges
175 g (6 oz) wholemeal bread
(about 4 large slices), thinly
sliced
50 g (2 oz) low fat soft cheese

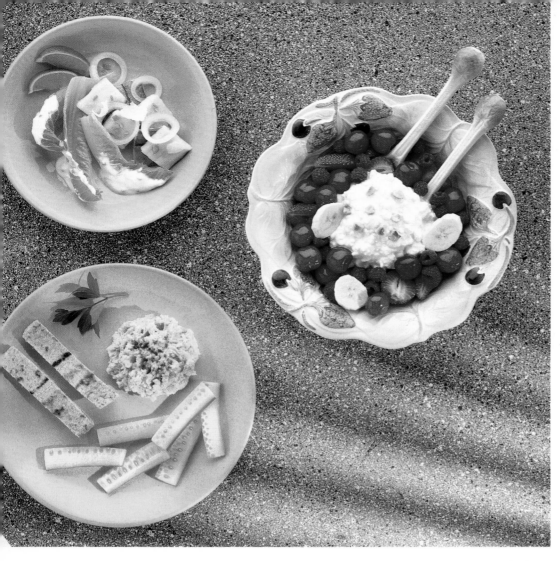

PREPARATION TIME:
15 minutes, plus standing and chilling
COOKING TIME:
about 1 hour 10 minutes
CALORIES PER SERVING:
about 365 (1515 kilojoules)

A low-calorie variation of a traditional Middle Eastern dish, made without the oil that is usually included.

1. Place the chick peas in a saucepan, cover with water, bring to the boil and simmer for 2–3 minutes. Turn off the heat and leave the pan to stand for 2–3 hours.
2. Drain the water and replace with fresh water to cover. Bring to the boil, cover and simmer for about 1 hour or until the chick peas are tender.
3. Place the sesame seeds in an ungreased heavy-based frying pan and stir over a low heat for 2–3 minutes until they begin to 'jump'. Grind in an electric coffee mill or with a mortar and pestle.
4. Transfer the seeds to a liquidizer and add the garlic, 2 tablespoons of the lemon juice, coriander, oil, pepper and salt. Blend.
5. Add the cooked chick peas and blend with enough cooking water to make a smooth, thick pureé. You will probably have to do this in batches.
6. Transfer to a bowl then stir in the cheese by hand.
7. Taste and add the remaining lemon juice, salt and pepper to taste. Refrigerate for a few hours or overnight if you can.
8. To serve, transfer the mixture to a flat dish and sprinkle with paprika. Arrange the pitta bread and vegetable strips on a second platter and garnish with lovage or celery leaves. Serve with the hummus.

PREPARATION TIME:
10 minutes, plus chilling
CALORIES PER SERVING:
about 290 (1200 kilojoules)
250 (1020 kilojoules) without coconut

A cross between Central American and Pacific fish recipes, this will surprise you if you dislike the idea of eating fish that hasn't been cooked with heat: here, the citrus juice does the job.

1. Place the fish, citrus juice, onions, chilli and coconut (if using) in a deep glass or stainless steel bowl. Refrigerate for at least 3 hours, turning from time to time.
2. Drain off the citrus juice and mix it with the yogurt or smetana, chives, ginger and salt.
3. Divide the lettuce leaves between 4 plates and top with the fish mixture. Spoon the dressing mixture over the lettuce. Place 2 lime wedges on each plate. Spread each slice of bread thinly with the soft cheese and serve with the ceviche.

Hummus with Pitta Bread and Vegetable Strips

175 g (6 oz) chick peas, washed
40 g (1½ oz) sesame seeds
2 garlic cloves, peeled (optional)
4 tablespoons lemon juice
½–1 teaspoon ground coriander
1 tablespoon olive oil
pinch of pepper
pinch of salt
175 g (6 oz) low fat soft cheese
To serve:
paprika, to dust
100 g (4 oz) wholemeal pitta bread, toasted and cut into fingers
100 g (4 oz) carrots, cut into strips (optional)
225 g (8 oz) cucumber, cut into strips
sprigs of fresh lovage or celery leaves, to garnish

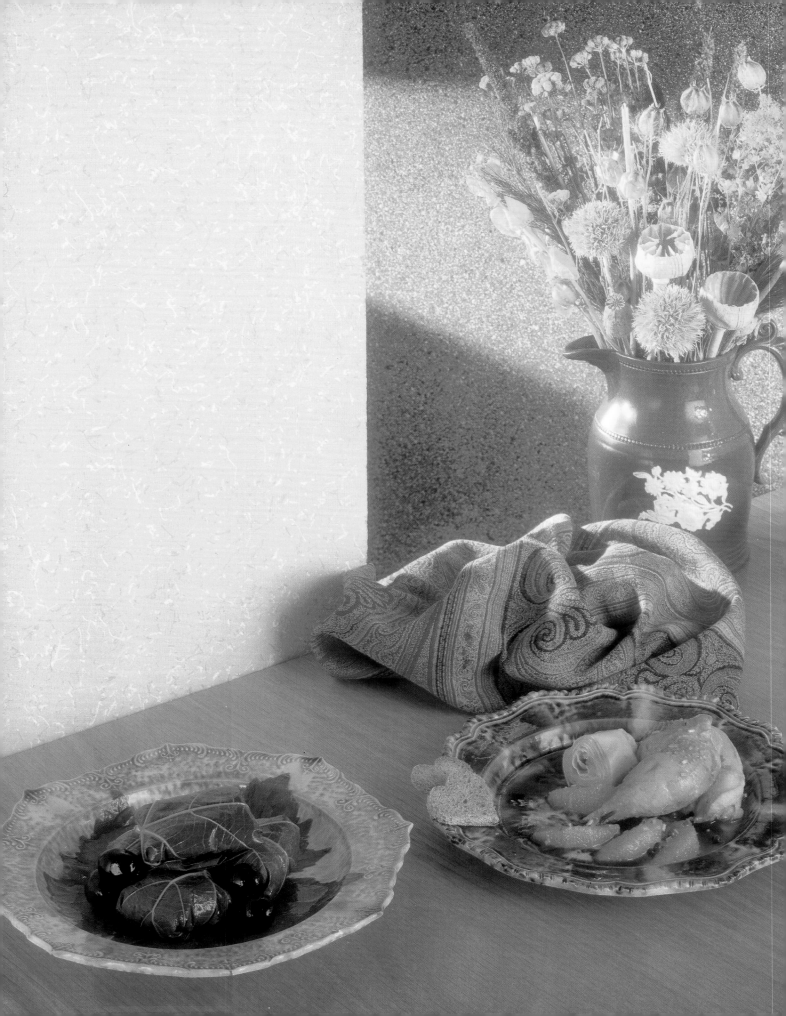

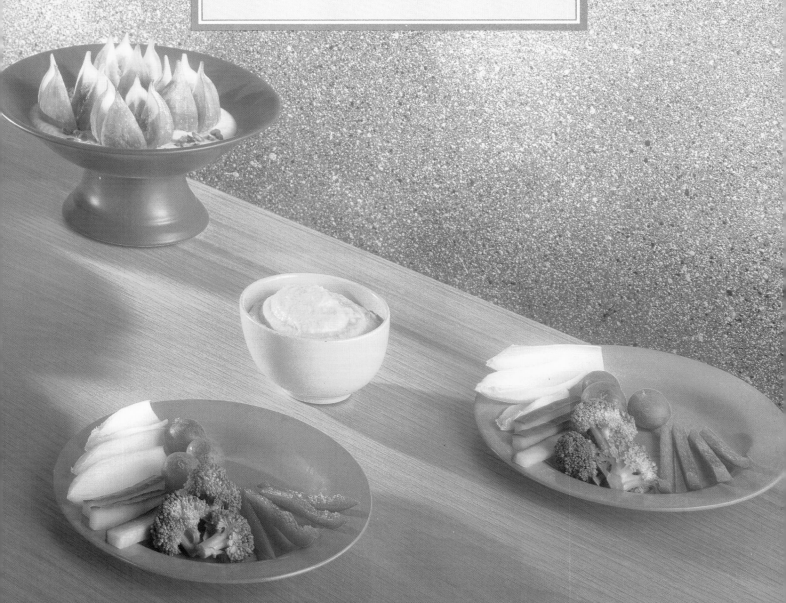

AUTUMN

SEPTEMBER

Celebration Dinner for Ten

It does not matter what you are celebrating, a wedding anniversary, a birthday, an engagement or someone's good fortune, the delicate summery cake will say all you want for the occasion.

Spinach and Black-eyed Beans

750 g (1½ lb) fresh spinach
350 g (12 oz) black-eyed beans
2 onions, peeled and chopped
1 tablespoon olive oil
150 ml (¼ pint) white wine
150 ml (¼ pint) white wine vinegar
1 teaspoon ground cinnamon
salt
freshly ground black pepper

PREPARATION TIME:
5 minutes
COOKING TIME:
1½ hours
CALORIES PER PORTION:
140 (585 kilojoules)

1. Wash and coarsely chop the spinach, add the beans to it in a saucepan, cover with cold water and bring to the boil. Cook gently for about 15 minutes, then drain, cover again with cold water, bring back to the boil and cook gently for 15 minutes.
2. Repeat the process twice, then continue to simmer until the beans are tender, approximately 45 minutes.
3. Fry the onions in the oil until translucent.
4. Thoroughly drain the spinach and beans and add them to the onions, pour in the wine and vinegar, stir in the cinnamon and plenty of salt and pepper.
5. Serve tepid or cold.

Fancy Dress Chicken

2 courgettes
2 bunches spring onions
2 small red peppers, cored and seeded
½ summer cabbage such as drumhead
350 g (12 oz) fresh mushrooms
salt
2 chickens, about 2 kg (4½ lb) each
1 tablespoon chopped fresh thyme, sage and parsley, mixed
1 garlic clove, peeled and chopped
1 tablespoon lemon juice
freshly ground black pepper
2 sprigs each thyme, sage and parsley (or any combination of your choice)

PREPARATION TIME:
25 minutes
COOKING TIME:
1½–2 hours
OVEN TEMPERATURE:
220°C, 425°F, Gas Mark 7
CALORIES PER PORTION:
250 (1040 kilojoules)

1. Cut all the vegetables into strips about twice the width and length of

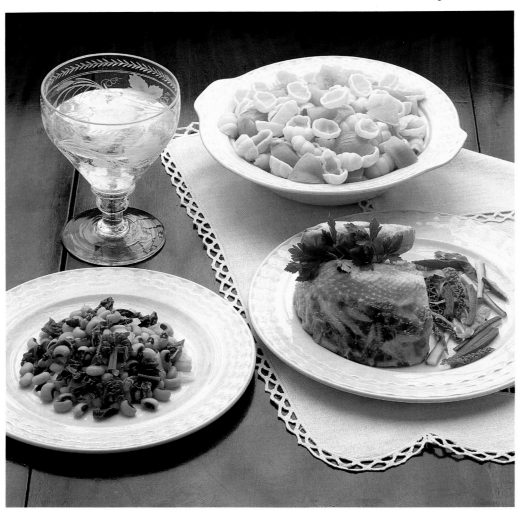

matchsticks and place them together in a bowl; sprinkle with salt and cover with boiling water. Leave to stand just long enough to soften the vegetables and cool them enough to handle.

2. Put your hand into the neck cavity of each chicken and very carefully loosen the skin covering the breast with your fingers so you can slip your hand all over the breast quite freely. Take great care not to tear the skin.

3. Strain the vegetables and combine with the chopped herbs, garlic, lemon juice and pepper.

4. Stuff the chickens with the vegetable mixture under the loosened skin, completely covering the breasts and filling the neck ends, then fill the body cavities. Close the necks with a cocktail stick or two. Push the "parson's noses" up into the cavity openings and secure with string, making sure the legs are tight to the bodies.

5. Place a double layer of greased foil over the breasts. Stand in a roasting dish, pour in enough water to cover a quarter of the way up the sides of the dish and surround with the sprigs of fresh herbs.

6. Cook in a preheated oven for 1½ hours, then remove the foil and brown the breasts. Continue cooking if necessary. Test by piercing the fattest part of the thigh; the liquid should be clear and not pink if the birds are cooked.

7. To serve, cut the string after letting the birds rest out of the oven for at least 8–10 minutes. Cut the chickens into quarters, with the aid of poultry shears if you like. Halve the quarters to serve 10.

Green Tomato and Pasta Salad

1 kg (2 lb) green tomatoes
6 cloves garlic, peeled and sliced, not too thinly
2 tablespoons olive oil
450 g (1 lb) cooked pasta shells
1 tablespoon white wine vinegar
salt
freshly ground black pepper

PREPARATION TIME:
8–10 minutes
COOKING TIME:
10–12 minutes
CALORIES PER PORTION:
95 (400 kilojoules)

The large really fleshy green tomatoes are best for this dish.

1. Cut the tomatoes into small chunks removing as much seed pulp as possible.

2. Fry the garlic in the olive oil until lightly burnt. Add the tomatoes, cover and cook for about 6–8 minutes over a gentle heat.

3. Combine the cooked pasta with the tomatoes and garlic and season with the vinegar, salt and pepper. Serve cold or tepid.

Celebration Gâteau

Sponge:
4 eggs, separated
75 g (3 oz) granulated sugar
75 g (3 oz) plain flour, sieved
1 teaspoon finely grated lemon rind
Filling:
300 g (11 oz) very mild low fat soft cheese
450 g (1 lb) September raspberries
25 g (1 oz) caster sugar
To decorate:
15 g (½ oz) icing sugar
fresh flowers (see right)
1 egg white
caster sugar

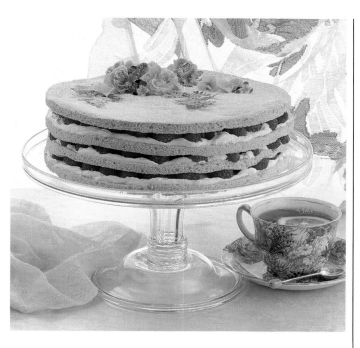

OPPOSITE, CLOCKWISE FROM BOTTOM Spinach and black-eyed beans; Green tomato and pasta salad; Fancy dress chicken ABOVE Celebration gâteau

PREPARATION TIME:
1 hour
COOKING TIME:
28 minutes
OVEN TEMPERATURE:
180°C, 350°F, Gas Mark 4
CALORIES PER PORTION:
140 (585 kilojoules)

1. Grease and line 2 × 23 cm (9 inch) sandwich tins with non-stick silicone paper.

2. Cream the egg yolks with the sugar until very light, frothy and creamy.

3. Whip the egg whites until stiff and stir into the creamed yolks. Fold in the flour and lemon rind.

4. Spread ¼ of the mixture in each sandwich tin. Spread it very thinly and evenly – this cannot be rushed.

5. Bake in a preheated oven for 7 minutes. Turn out, with the aid of a spatula, on to a flat surface to cool. Repeat the process so that you have 4 thin sponges.

6. Place one of the sponges on a cake-stand or large plate. Spread over a layer of soft cheese. Arrange some of the raspberries on top and sprinkle with a little of the sugar. Repeat the process with the remaining sponges, finishing with a layer of sponge. Sift the icing sugar over the top layer.

7. Prepare the flowers as follows. Choose small flowers that do not come from bulbs. Summer jasmine, polyanthus (in its second flower by now), tiny roses, sprigs of herbs such as sweet cicely, rosemary, mint and basil work well; miniature pansies look good too. Lightly beat the egg white and paint the flower or leaf all over with it, then dredge with sugar, set on a wire rack on non-stick silicone paper in a warm place such as the airing cupboard to dry for several hours. Arrange on top of the cake at the last minute.

Hors d'oeuvres and Light Meals

Vegetable Salad with Tarragon Mayonnaise

4 medium carrots, peeled and
  cut into thin strips
225 g (8 oz) French beans,
  trimmed
2 leeks, cleaned and cut into
  rounds
6 tablespoons unsweetened
  orange juice
3 tablespoons olive oil
1 garlic clove, peeled and
  crushed
salt
freshly ground black pepper
1 × 425 g (15 oz) can black-
  eyed beans, drained and
  rinsed
175 g (6 oz) Brussels sprouts,
  trimmed, washed and finely
  shredded
10–12 good-shaped spinach
  leaves
sprigs of fresh tarragon, to
  garnish

Tarragon mayonnaise:
2 egg yolks
1 tablespoon lemon juice
150 ml (¼ pint) olive oil
1 garlic clove, peeled and
  crushed
½ teaspoon French mustard
1½ tablespoons chopped fresh
  tarragon
4 tablespoons plain
  unsweetened yogurt

1. Steam the strips of carrot, sliced beans and leek rounds until just tender – the vegetables should still have a 'bite' to them. Allow to cool.
2. Mix the orange juice with the olive oil, garlic and salt and pepper to taste; toss the black-eyed beans and the Brussels sprouts in the orange dressing.
3. To make the tarragon mayonnaise, beat the egg yolks with the lemon juice; whisk in the olive oil in a fine trickle. Blend in the garlic, mustard, tarragon, yogurt and salt and pepper to taste.
4. Arrange a bed of spinach leaves on each serving plate; spoon the black-eyed beans and shredded sprouts on top.
5. Arrange the carrots, leeks and beans around the salad.
6. Garnish with sprigs of tarragon and serve as a complete light meal, accompanied by the tarragon mayonnaise.

PREPARATION TIME:
45 minutes
COOKING TIME:
8–10 minutes
CALORIES PER PORTION:
250 (990 kilojoules)

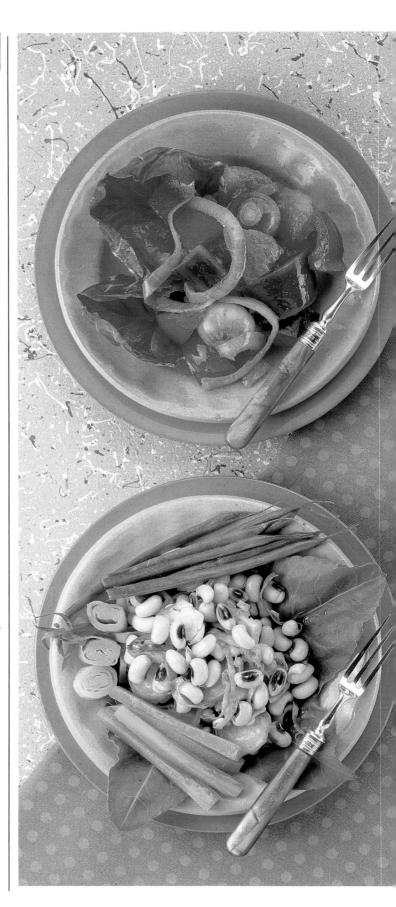

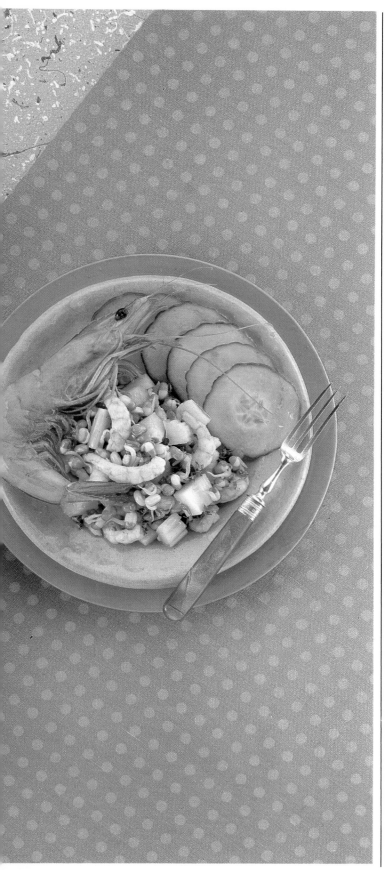

Ratatouille

4 tablespoons olive oil
1 large onion, peeled and
  thinly sliced
2 garlic cloves, peeled and
  crushed
450 g (1 lb) tomatoes,
  skinned, seeded and chopped
4 tablespoons red wine
1 tablespoon tomato purée
1 green pepper, seeded and
  roughly chopped
1 red pepper, seeded and
  roughly chopped
1 medium aubergine, cubed
12 small pickling onions,
  peeled
salt
freshly ground black pepper
radicchio leaves, to garnish

PREPARATION TIME:
about 15 minutes
COOKING TIME:
15–20 minutes
CALORIES PER PORTION:
200 (840 kilojoules)

1. Heat 2 tablespoons of
olive oil in a deep frying
pan and fry the onion and
garlic gently for 3–4
minutes.
2. Add the tomatoes, red
wine and tomato purée;
simmer until the tomatoes
are soft and pulpy. Add the
remaining olive oil.
3. Add the peppers,
aubergine, onions and salt
and pepper to taste; cover
and simmer gently until
the vegetables are tender
but still have a 'bite' to
them.
4. Serve warm, on small
plates, garnished with
radicchio leaves.

Mung Bean and Prawn Salad

3 tablespoons olive oil
3 tablespoons lemon juice
1 garlic clove, peeled and
  crushed
2 tablespoons finely chopped
  fresh parsley
salt
freshly ground black pepper
3 celery sticks, finely chopped
225 g (8 oz) mung bean
  sprouts
175 g (6 oz) peeled prawns
To garnish:
thinly sliced cucumber
4 cooked Mediterranean
  prawns

PREPARATION TIME:
about 15 minutes
CALORIES PER PORTION:
170 (710 kilojoules)

Mung bean sprouts are
available from
supermarkets and health
food shops.

1. Mix the olive oil with
the lemon juice, garlic,
parsley and salt and pepper
to taste.
2. Mix the celery, mung
sprouts and peeled prawns
together; stir in the oil and
lemon dressing.
3. Spoon the prepared
salad on to small serving
plates; arrange a border of
overlapping cucumber
slices around each one and
garnish with a
Mediterranean prawn.

CLOCKWISE FROM RIGHT Mung
bean and prawn salad; Vegetable salad
with tarragon mayonnaise; Ratatouille

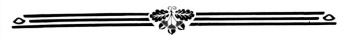

SEPTEMBER

Main Courses

Scallops in Light Curry Sauce

16 large shelled scallops
2 tablespoons Pernod
2 tablespoons dry white wine
1 tablespoon chopped parsley
salt
freshly ground black pepper
3 spring onions, chopped
20 g (¾ oz) butter
1 tablespoon olive oil
1 dessertspoon seasoned flour
2 teaspoons mild curry
  powder
300 ml (½ pint) chicken stock
1 tablespoon peach chutney
thin lime wedges, to garnish

PREPARATION TIME:
15 minutes, plus chilling
COOKING TIME:
about 7 minutes
CALORIES PER PORTION:
220 (920 kilojoules)

1. Halve each scallop
horizontally; put in a
shallow dish with the
Pernod, wine, parsley and
salt and pepper. Cover and
chill for 2 hours.
2. Lift the scallops out of
their marinade and drain,
reserving the marinade.
3. Fry the chopped spring
onions gently in the butter
and oil for 2–3 minutes.
4. Dust the scallops *lightly*
with seasoned flour and fry
gently for about 2 minutes.
5. Stir in the curry powder,
and then add the chicken
stock, marinade and the
peach chutney; simmer
gently for 2 minutes until
the scallops are just tender.
6. Serve immediately,
with rice and lime wedges.

Sautéed Kidneys with Vegetable Julienne

12 lambs' kidneys, skinned,
  halved and cored
1 dessertspoon seasoned flour
1 small onion, chopped
1 tablespoon olive oil
3 medium carrots, peeled and
  cut into julienne strips
2 leeks, cleaned and cut into
  julienne strips
100 g (4 oz) button
  mushrooms, thinly sliced
150 ml (¼ pint) beef stock
4 tablespoons dry sherry
salt
freshly ground black pepper
julienne strips of carrot and
  leek, blanched, to garnish

PREPARATION TIME:
20 minutes
COOKING TIME:
about 20 minutes
CALORIES PER PORTION:
200 (880 kilojoules)

1. Dust the lambs' kidneys
lightly with seasoned flour.
2. Fry the onion gently in
the oil for 3–4 minutes;
add the kidneys and fry
until sealed on all sides.
3. Add the strips of carrot
and leek and the sliced
mushrooms and fry
together for 1 minute.
4. Stir in the stock and
sherry and bring to the
boil; add salt and pepper to
taste, and simmer gently
until the kidneys are just
tender (12–15 minutes).
Take care not to overcook,
as they quickly go rubbery.
5. Serve, garnished with
strips of carrot and leek.

Nut-Stuffed Marrow

1 medium marrow
1 large onion, peeled and
  finely chopped
1 garlic clove, peeled and
  crushed
2 tablespoons olive oil
225 g (8 oz) fresh spinach,
  cooked and drained
100 g (4 oz) button
  mushrooms, finely chopped
50 g (2 oz) chopped pine
  kernels
25 g (1 oz) chopped toasted
  almonds
2 hard-boiled eggs, chopped
salt
freshly ground black pepper

PREPARATION TIME:
20 minutes
COOKING TIME:
45 minutes–1 hour
OVEN TEMPERATURE:
180°C, 350°F, Gas Mark 4
CALORIES PER PORTION:
290 (1210 kilojoules)

1. Cut a slice from each
end of the marrow, about
1 cm (½ inch) thick. Slice
the marrow in half
horizontally and scoop out
all the centre seeds.
2. Fry the onion and garlic
gently in the olive oil for
4–5 minutes; mix with the
remaining ingredients, to
make a firm stuffing.
3. Pack the stuffing tightly
into the marrow halves
and wrap each half
securely in foil.
4. Bake in a preheated
oven for about 45
minutes–1 hour until the
marrow is tender.
5. Serve hot, cut into thick
slices, accompanied by low
calorie mayonnaise if
liked.

CLOCKWISE FROM RIGHT Nut-
stuffed marrow; Scallops in light curry
sauce; Sautéed kidneys with vegetable
julienne

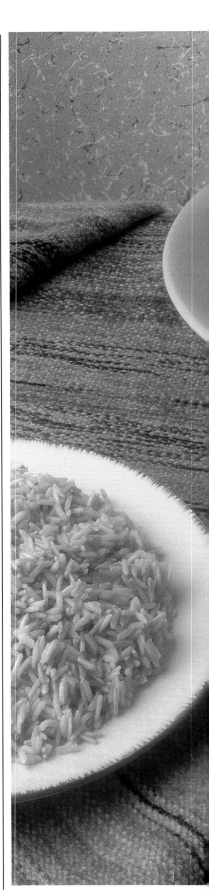

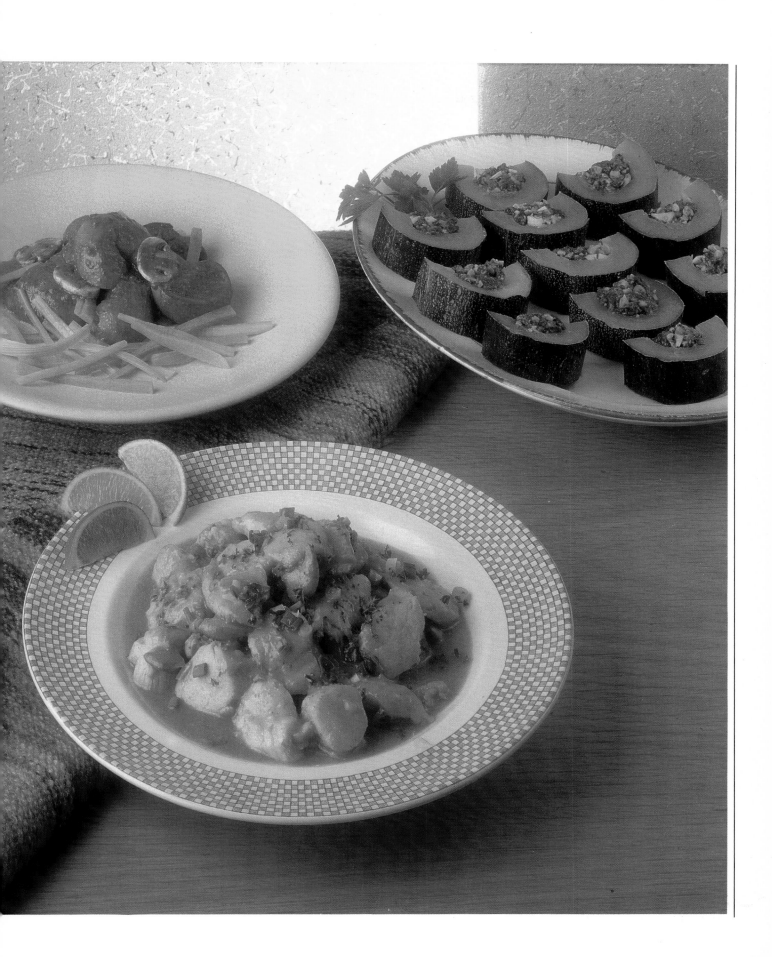

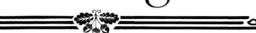

SEPTEMBER

Puddings

Melon Ice Cream

1 medium melon (Ogen or
  Charentais)
300 ml (½ pint) plain
  unsweetened yogurt
artificial sweetener (optional)
small melon balls, to decorate

PREPARATION TIME:
20–25 minutes, plus freezing
CALORIES PER PORTION:
65 (270 kilojoules)

1. Halve the melon and
scoop out all the seeds;
scoop the melon flesh into
the liquidizer, and blend
until smooth.
2. Mix the melon purée
with the yogurt and add
artificial sweetener to
taste.
3. Transfer the melon and
yogurt mixture to a
shallow container, and
freeze until firm.
4. Serve the melon ice
cream in scoops, decorated
with melon balls.

Sliced Figs with Lemon Sauce

8 plump ripe figs
2 tablespoons lemon juice
150 ml (¼ pint) unsweetened
  apple purée
grated rind of ½ lemon
3 tablespoons plain
  unsweetened yogurt
artificial sweetener
1 tablespoon chopped
  pistachio nuts
4 twists of lemon peel, to
  decorate (optional)

PREPARATION TIME:
15–20 minutes
CALORIES PER PORTION:
110 (460 kilojoules)

1. Cut each fig into 4
wedges. (Alternatively, the
figs can be sliced, provided
they are not too soft.)
Sprinkle the cut figs with
lemon juice.
2. Mix the apple purée
with the lemon rind and
yogurt; add artificial
sweetener to taste and half
the chopped pistachios.
3. Spoon a pool of the
lemon and pistachio sauce
on to each of 4 small plates
and arrange the pieces of
fig decoratively on top.
4. Sprinkle with the
remaining pistachio nuts
and decorate with twists of
lemon peel if liked.

CLOCKWISE FROM LEFT Sliced figs
with lemon sauce; Melon ice cream;
Iced stuffed apples

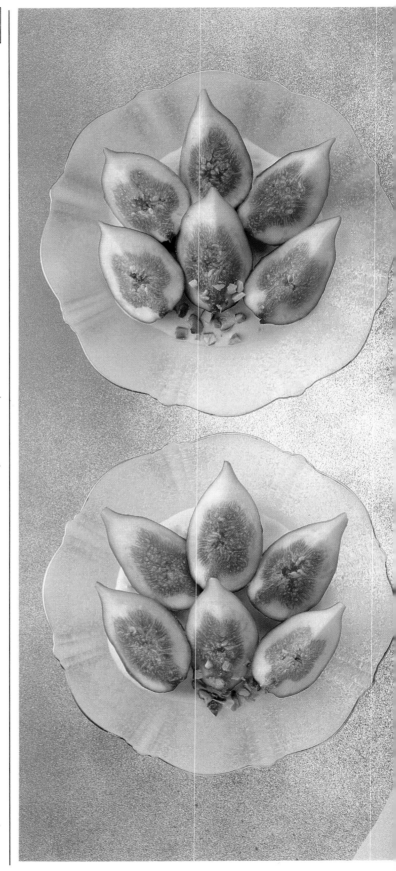

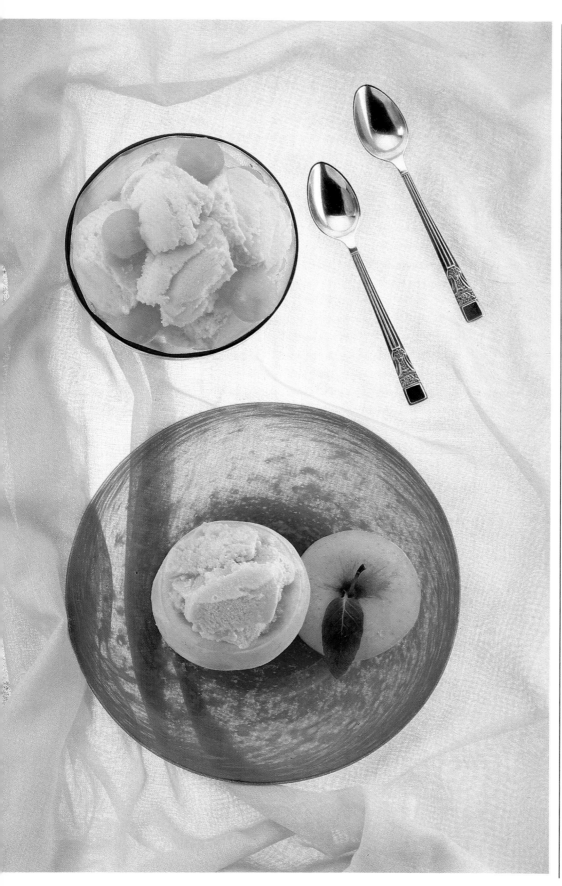

Iced Stuffed Apples

*2 medium cooking apples,
   peeled, cored and sliced
4 tablespoons lemon juice
2 tablespoons brandy
2 egg yolks
3 tablespoons plain
   unsweetened yogurt
4 red or green dessert apples
1 egg white
2 tablespoons sultanas*

PREPARATION TIME:
35 minutes, plus freezing
COOKING TIME:
5–6 minutes
CALORIES PER PORTION:
60 (250 kilojoules)

1. Stew the cooking apples
with half the lemon juice
in a covered pan until they
are tender.
2. Beat in the brandy and
egg yolks and allow to
cool.
3. Mix the yogurt with the
cooled apple purée; pour
into a shallow container,
and freeze until firm
around the edges.
4. Cut a thin slice from the
stalk end of each dessert
apple, about 1 cm (½ inch)
thick and reserve for lids.
Carefully hollow out the
centre flesh and core,
leaving a 'shell' about 5
mm (¼ inch) thick. Brush
inside with the remaining
lemon juice.
5. Tip the semi-frozen
apple mixture into a bowl
and beat until smooth.
6. Whisk the egg white
until stiff but not dry; fold
lightly but thoroughly into
the apple mixture,
together with the sultanas.
7. Spoon the apple mixture
into the hollow apples, and
replace the lids. Open
freeze until firm.
8. Remove the frozen filled
apples from the freezer a
few minutes before serving
to allow the centres to
soften slightly.

SEPTEMBER

Dinner Party for Six

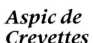

Aspic de Crevettes

600 ml (1 pint) aspic
2 tablespoons sherry
small handful feathery fennel
  leaves
1 small cucumber
salt
3 hard-boiled eggs
1 teaspoon mild curry powder
3 teaspoons lemon juice
vinegar
white pepper
1 red pepper, seeded, and cut
  into matchstick strips
36 peeled prawns

PREPARATION TIME:
20–30 minutes, plus chilling
CALORIES PER PORTION:
100 (420 kilojoules)

1. Make up the aspic,
incorporating the sherry in
the liquid, and snip in
some fennel leaves. Pour a
little into the bottom of 6
individual shallow
ramekins and allow to set.
2. Slice the cucumber
thinly, sprinkle with salt
and set aside.
3. Slice the hard-boiled
eggs in half widthways.
Cut the end piece off each
egg and discard it. Take out
the yolks and mash them,
adding a pinch or two of
curry powder and the
lemon juice. Add salt to
taste.
4. Put the mashed yolks
back into the whites and
smooth them over.

5. Pour boiling water over
the cucumber, drain,
sprinkle with vinegar and
white pepper and mix
well.
6. Arrange 5–6
overlapping cucumber
slices around the inside
edge of each dish, then
place one filled egg half,
yolk side upward, in each.
Arrange 5–6 strips of red
pepper and 5–6 prawns
alternately around the
edge, in between the
cucumber and the egg.
Place a small sprig of
fennel on each egg yolk,
pour enough aspic to cover
into each ramekin and chill
until set.
7. Chill until the last
moment, then turn out.

Stir-Fried Liver and Fennel

750 g (1½ lb) calves' liver,
  trimmed
1 tablespoon oil
1 large fennel bulb, finely
  sliced into thin strips
3 garlic cloves, peeled and
  chopped
3 tablespoons tomato purée
3 tablespoons red wine
salt
freshly ground black pepper
1 tablespoon chopped parsley

PREPARATION TIME:
10 minutes
COOKING TIME:
10–15 minutes
CALORIES PER PORTION:
230 (960 kilojoules)

You will need to cook this
dish at the last minute, but
you can prepare everything
ahead of time as the
cooking is brief and easy. A
wok is ideal for it, but a
large heavy frying pan can
be used.

1. Cut the liver into 1 cm
(½ inch) wide strips.
2. Heat the oil and add the
fennel and garlic. Stir and
cook for a few minutes
over a medium to high
heat.
3. As soon as the fennel
begins to colour slightly,
add the liver and stir
continuously.
4. After 1 minute add the
tomato purée and wine,
bring to boiling point,
simmer for 2 minutes, then
remove from the heat. Add
salt and pepper to taste and
stir in the parsley.
5. Serve with rice, or
steamed potatoes and
salad.

Fresh Blackberries with Hazelnut Cheese

750 g (1½ lb) freshly picked
  wild blackberries
1 tablespoon soft dark brown
  sugar
1–2 teaspoons Angostura
  bitters
50 g (2 oz) hazelnuts
1 teaspoon caster sugar
6 Petit Suisse cheeses

PREPARATION TIME:
10 minutes
COOKING TIME:
3 minutes
CALORIES PER PORTION:
140 (590 kilojoules)

1. Sort through the
blackberries and discard
any that look hard or even
slightly red. Mix the brown
sugar and Angostura
bitters with the remaining
blackberries.
2. In a frying pan toast the
hazelnuts and add the
caster sugar when they
have coloured. Shake the
pan continuously to coat
the nuts in the now
melting and caramelized
sugar. Set aside to cool.
3. When cold, crush or
grind the caramel-coated
nuts, then spread them out
on a large sheet of
greaseproof paper.
4. Roll each Petit Suisse in
the crushed nuts, gently
pressing the nuts on to the
surface. As each cheese is
covered, transfer it to a
plate in the refrigerator to
set slightly.
5. Just before serving,
place the balls in individual
serving bowls and
surround each one with
blackberries.

CLOCKWISE FROM LEFT Aspic de
crevettes; Fresh blackberries with
hazelnut cheese; Stir-fried liver and
fennel

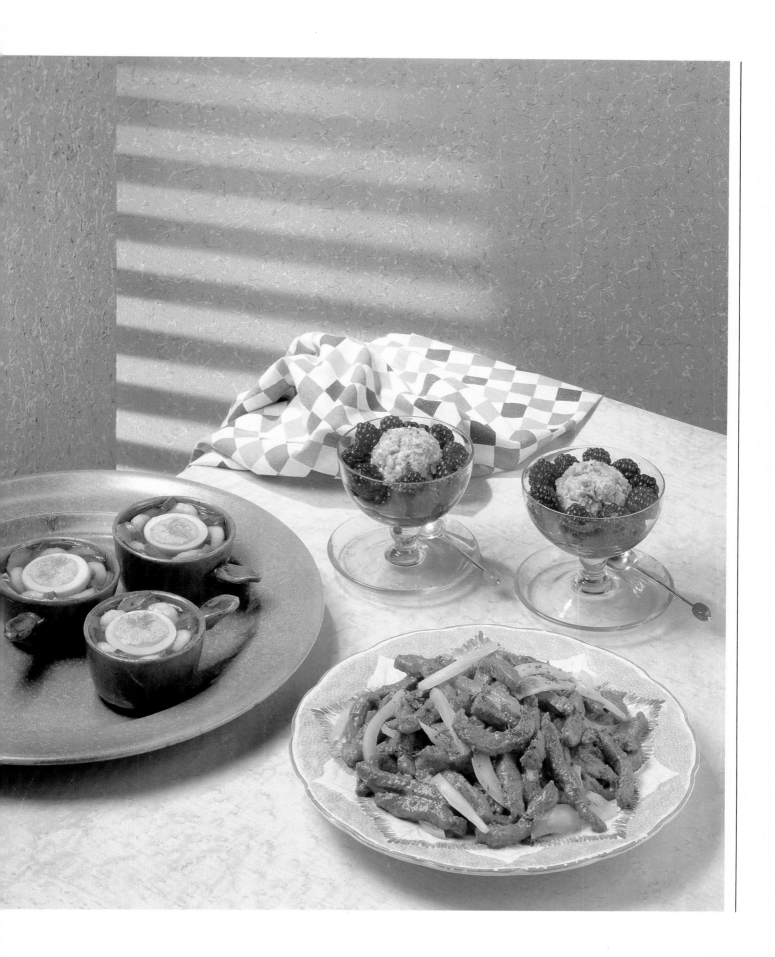

OCTOBER
Halloween Party for Twelve

An unusual pumpkin salad and flaming apples bring to this menu a touch of Hallowe'en atmosphere without evoking too contrived a spooky mood.

Pumpkin Salad

2 small pumpkins, washed
4 garlic cloves, peeled
salt
25 g (1 oz) butter, melted
lemon juice
Filling:
225 g (8 oz) rice, cooked
225 g (8 oz) peas, cooked
225 g (8 oz) white cabbage,
    shredded and blanched
1 red pepper, cored, seeded
    and chopped
1 fennel bulb, chopped
1 Jerusalem artichoke,
    washed, scraped and grated
4 ripe tomatoes, skinned,
    seeded and chopped
50 g (2 oz) sultanas
1 small apple, grated
1 tablespoon chopped parsley
1 teaspoon caraway seeds
2 tablespoons wine vinegar
1 tablespoon olive oil
coarsely ground black pepper

PREPARATION TIME:
40 minutes
COOKING TIME:
50 minutes
OVEN TEMPERATURE:
180°C, 350°F, Gas Mark 4
CALORIES PER PORTION:
130 (545 kilojoules)

1. Cut off the tops of the pumpkins, about one-quarter of the way down. Scoop out seeds and pulp.
2. Rub the insides of both with a cut clove of garlic and sprinkle with salt. Put 1 garlic clove in each, replace the 'lids' and bake in a preheated oven for 35 minutes, then brush the insides with the butter and a little more salt and continue to bake for a further 15 minutes.
3. Scoop out about half the pumpkin flesh, mash 3 tablespoons of it with the cooked garlic, crush the remaining 2 cloves and combine. Sprinkle with a little lemon juice and spread inside the pumpkins.
4. When the pumpkins are cold, combine all the filling ingredients thoroughly in a bowl and spoon them in.

Brodetto di Pesce

1.75 kg (4 lb) cleaned fish and
    seafood eg. sole, red mullet,
    monkfish, prepared squid,
    sardines, clams, cooked
    shelled mussels, giant
    prawns (see below)
2 tablespoons olive oil
3 onions, peeled and coarsely
    chopped
6 red peppers, cored and
    quartered
1–2 red chillies, or to taste,
    seeded and left whole
3 × 400g (14 oz) cans
    tomatoes
250 ml (8 fl oz) red wine
    vinegar
1½ tablespoons anchovy
    essence
salt
freshly ground black pepper
4–8 cooked unshelled
    mussels, to garnish
    (optional)

PREPARATION TIME:
about 1 hour
COOKING TIME:
about 40 minutes
CALORIES PER PORTION:
150 (630 kilojoules)

This is a version of a traditional fish soup from the Abruzzi. It is more a casserole of fish than a soup, a complete and wonderful meal, ideal for a large gathering.

1. Cut the fish into bite-size pieces. Leave the shellfish whole.
2. Heat the oil in a flameproof casserole or a large frying pan. Sweat the onions, peppers and chillies, covered, until the peppers are really soft. Remove the peppers with a perforated spoon and push them through the finest disc of a vegetable mill or a fine sieve. Return them to the pan.
3. Seed the tomatoes by pushing them through the vegetable mill and add them to the pan. Stir, then add the vinegar and anchovy essence.
4. Bring the mixture to the boil and, after about 5 minutes, add all the fish except the seafood. Cook briskly for 10 minutes, then add the remaining items.
5. Cook for a further 5 minutes, or remove from the heat and reheat and cook for the final minutes just before serving. Adjust the seasoning with salt and plenty of freshly ground pepper. Serve, garnished with unshelled mussels.

CLOCKWISE FROM TOP Pommes flambées au Calvados; Jacket potatoes with herbed cottage cheese; Brodetto di pesce; Pumpkin salad

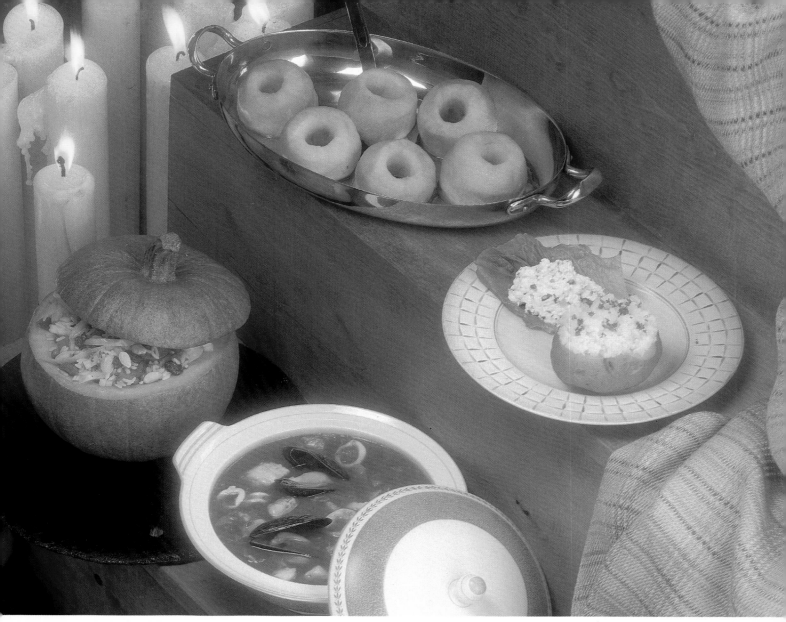

Jacket Potatoes with Herbed Cottage Cheese

12 medium floury potatoes,
  scrubbed
salt
1 kg (2 lb) cottage cheese
1 tablespoon finely chopped
  fresh sage
2 teaspoons lemon juice
1 teaspoon green peppercorns
  in brine, crushed
To serve:
12 small crisp lettuce leaves
chopped fresh parsley

PREPARATION TIME:
15 minutes
COOKING TIME:
1 hour 10 minutes
OVEN TEMPERATURE:
230°C, 450°F, Gas Mark 8
CALORIES PER PORTION:
210 (880 kilojoules)

1. Rub each potato all over
with salt and pierce. Bake
in a preheated oven for
60–70 minutes.
2. Push the cottage cheese
through a fine sieve and
mix in the sage, lemon
juice and peppercorns.
3. Cut off the top of each
potato, fluff up the insides
and sprinkle with parsley.
Serve the potatoes on
lettuce leaves accompanied
by the herbed cheese.

Pommes Flambées au Calvados

12 small cooking apples
1 tablespoon salt
50 g (2 oz) butter, melted
50 g (2 oz) caster sugar
3 tablespoons Calvados

PREPARATION TIME:
10 minutes
COOKING TIME:
45–50 minutes
OVEN TEMPERATURE:
160°C, 325°F, Gas Mark 3
CALORIES PER PORTION:
95 (400 kilojoules)

1. Peel and core the apples,
plunging them into a basin
of salted water to prevent
discoloration.

2. Dry the apples, then
pour a little cooled melted
butter into the palm of
your hand and rub it all
over them. Stand them in a
greased baking dish and
sprinkle the sugar over.
Bake in a preheated oven
for 45 minutes.
3. Bring the apples to the
table, sprinkle the
Calvados over, stand well
back and set alight. Serve
immediately.

OCTOBER

Hors d'oeuvres and Light Meals

Bean-Stuffed Tomatoes

1 × 425 g (15 oz) can red
  kidney beans, drained
1 small onion, peeled and
  finely chopped
2 tablespoons finely chopped
  blanched almonds
1 teaspoon chopped fresh sage
1 garlic clove, peeled and
  finely chopped
2 tablespoons wholemeal
  breadcrumbs
1 small parsnip, peeled and
  grated
salt
freshly ground black pepper
4 large Mediterranean or 8
  medium tomatoes
1 tablespoon olive oil

PREPARATION TIME:
20–25 minutes
COOKING TIME:
15–20 minutes
OVEN TEMPERATURE:
180°C, 350°F, Gas Mark 4
CALORIES PER PORTION:
270 (1130 kilojoules)

1. Mix the beans with the
onion, almonds, sage,
garlic, breadcrumbs, grated
parsnip and seasonings.
2. Cut the tops off the
tomatoes and carefully
hollow them out. Fill each
with the bean mixture.
3. Stand the stuffed
tomatoes upright in a
lightly greased ovenproof
dish. Brush with a little oil.
4. Bake in a preheated
oven for 15–20 minutes.

Mushrooms in Herbed Vinaigrette

2 tablespoons walnut oil
2 tablespoons tarragon
  vinegar
4 tablespoons dry white wine
1 garlic clove, peeled and
  crushed
salt
freshly ground black pepper
1/2 teaspoon grated orange
  peel
1 tablespoon chopped fresh
  tarragon
1 tablespoon chopped parsley
225 g (8 oz) button
  mushrooms
2 pieces wholemeal pitta
  bread, cut into fingers

PREPARATION TIME:
5 minutes, plus chilling
COOKING TIME:
about 15 minutes
CALORIES PER PORTION:
140 (585kilojoules)

1. Put the walnut oil,
vinegar, wine and garlic
into a shallow pan and add
salt and pepper to taste;
simmer for 3 minutes.
2. Add the orange peel,
tarragon, parsley and
mushrooms; cover and
simmer for 8 minutes.
3. Pour the mushrooms
and their juices into a
shallow dish and allow to
cool. Cover and chill for 4
hours.
4. Serve with fingers of
warm pitta bread.

Jellied Grapefruit

2 large pink grapefruit,
  halved
300 ml (1/2 pint) unsweetened
  pineapple juice
150 ml (1/4 pint) unsweetened
  grapefruit juice
3 teaspoons gelatine
sprigs of fresh mint, to
  decorate

PREPARATION TIME:
40–45 minutes, plus chilling
CALORIES PER PORTION:
70 (295 kilojoules)

1. Carefully scoop out the
half segments of grapefruit,
making sure that they are
free from pith and
membrane. Remove all
remaining membrane and
loose pith from the
grapefruit shells.
2. Stand the 4 shells
upright on a tray or dish
and divide the segments
among them.
3. Combine the pineapple
and grapefruit juices. Put 2
tablespoons of the mixed
juices into a small bowl
with the gelatine; stand in
a pan of hot water and stir
until the gelatine has
dissolved.
4. Mix the dissolved
gelatine with the
remaining fruit juices;
pour carefully into each
grapefruit shell. Chill until
set.
5. Using a very sharp knife,
carefully cut each jellied
grapefruit half into 3
segments.
6. Arrange 3 segments on
each of 4 plates and
decorate with fresh mint.

CLOCKWISE FROM RIGHT Jellied
grapefruit; Mushrooms in herbed
vinaigrette; Bean-stuffed tomatoes

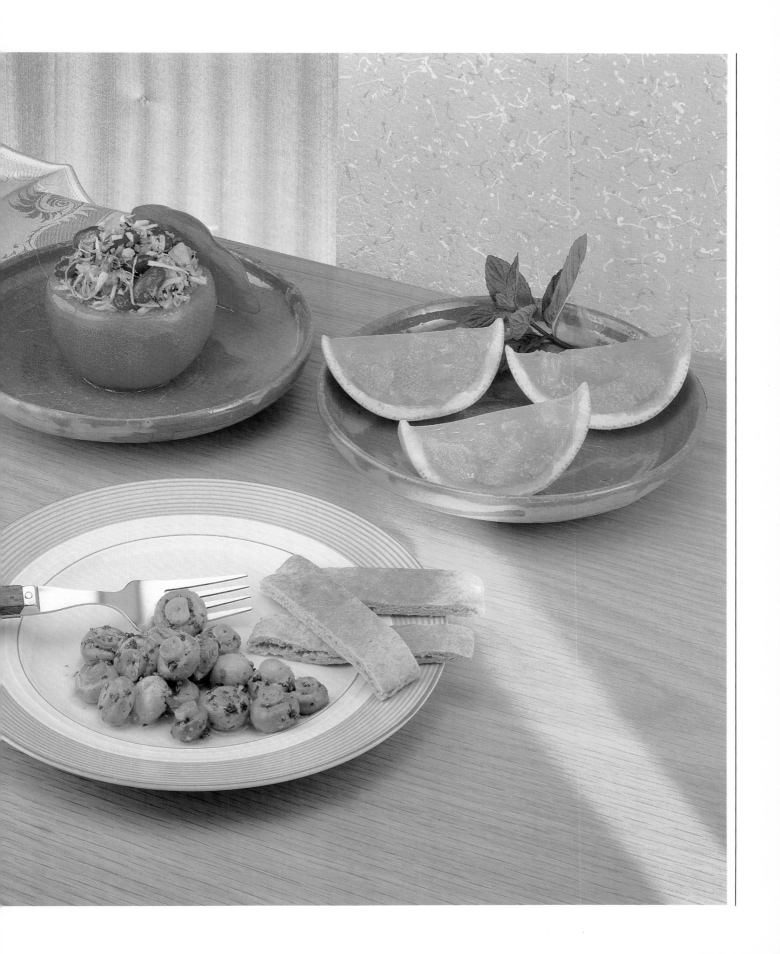

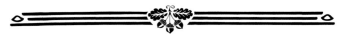

OCTOBER

Main Courses

Pheasant with Green Peppercorns

2 medium pheasants
12 tablespoons orange juice
1 garlic clove, peeled and crushed
1 tablespoon chopped chives
salt
2 teaspoons green peppercorns
150 ml (¼ pint) dry white wine
4 canned artichoke hearts
To garnish:
heart-shaped croûtons
peeled orange segments

PREPARATION TIME:
20–25 minutes, plus chilling
COOKING TIME:
about 30 minutes
CALORIES PER PORTION:
250 (1050 kilojoules)

1. Using a very sharp knife, remove the breasts and drumsticks from each bird.
2. Put the pheasant in a dish with the orange juice, garlic, chives and salt. Cover and chill 4 hours.
3. Transfer the pheasant and marinade to a frying pan. Add the peppercorns and the white wine and simmer for 15–20 minutes.
4. Add the artichoke hearts and simmer for a further 6–8 minutes, until the pheasant is just tender.
5. Remove the pheasant and artichoke hearts and keep warm.
6. Reduce the cooking juices slightly over a brisk heat; spoon over the pheasant and garnish with the croûtons and orange segments.

Curried Vegetables with Brown Rice

1 tablespoon olive oil
1 medium onion, peeled and finely chopped
1½ tablespoons Madras curry powder
1 garlic clove, peeled and crushed
6 tomatoes, skinned, seeded and chopped
1 thin slice fresh ginger, finely chopped
300 ml (½ pint) chicken stock
2 tablespoons lime juice
salt
freshly ground black pepper
8 pickling onions, peeled
225 g (8 oz) Brussels sprouts, trimmed
225 g (8 oz) carrots, peeled and cut into thin fingers
2 celery sticks, sliced
1 × 425 g (15 oz) can chick peas, drained
175 g (6 oz) soya bean sprouts
sprigs of fresh coriander, to garnish
To serve:
225 g (8 oz) cooked brown rice
3 ripe passion fruit, halved and pulp scooped out

PREPARATION TIME:
20 minutes
COOKING TIME:
about 25 minutes
CALORIES PER PORTION:
500 (2090 kilojoules)

1. Heat the oil and fry the onion gently for 3 minutes.
2. Add the curry powder and garlic and cook for 1 minute. Add the tomatoes, ginger, stock, lime juice and salt and pepper to taste. Bring to the boil and simmer for 5 minutes.
3. Add the pickling onions, sprouts, carrots and celery. Simmer, covered, for 10 minutes.
4. Add the chick peas and simmer for a further 5 minutes. Add the beansprouts and heat through.
5. Spoon on to 4 plates and garnish each one with coriander.
6. Place the rice in a serving dish and spoon the passion fruit pulp over. Serve immediately, with the curried vegetables.

Salmon and Cucumber Soufflé

225 g (8 oz) fresh salmon fillet
150 ml (¼ pint) dry white wine
1 bay leaf
salt
freshly ground black pepper
½ cucumber, coarsely grated
3 eggs, separated
20 g (¾ oz) butter
2 tablespoons flour
200 ml (⅓ pint) skimmed milk
2 teaspoons chopped fresh dill

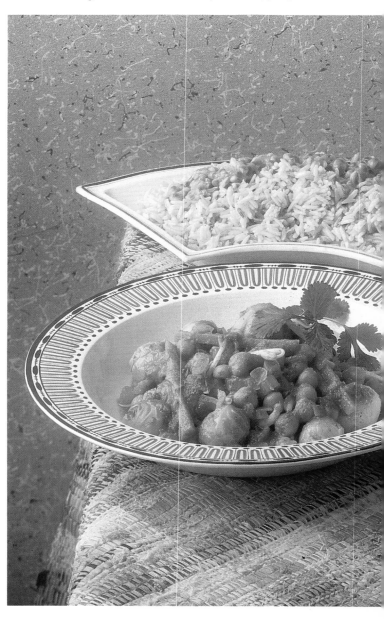

PREPARATION TIME:
50 minutes, plus cooling
COOKING TIME:
45–55 minutes
OVEN TEMPERATURE:
190°C, 375°F, Gas Mark 5
CALORIES PER PORTION:
270 (1130 kilojoules)

1. Lightly grease a 15 cm (6 inch) soufflé dish.
2. Put the salmon into a shallow pan with the wine, bay leaf and salt and pepper to taste. Poach gently until the salmon is just tender. Allow to cool in its cooking liquid.
3. Put the grated cucumber into a colander and sprinkle generously with salt; leave to drain for 20 minutes.
4. Flake the cooled salmon, reserving the poaching liquid.
5. Rinse the cucumber thoroughly then wring out in a clean teatowel. Beat the egg yolks together lightly.
6. Melt the butter, stir in the flour, and cook for 1 minute. Gradually stir in the skimmed milk and the strained salmon cooking liquid. Stir over a gentle heat until thickened. Stir in the flaked salmon, egg yolks and cucumber, season to taste with salt and pepper and add the dill.
7. Beat the egg whites until stiff but not dry; fold lightly but thoroughly into the cucumber and salmon sauce. Carefully pour into the soufflé dish.
8. Bake in a preheated oven for 30–40 minutes, until well risen, golden and just set. Serve immediately.

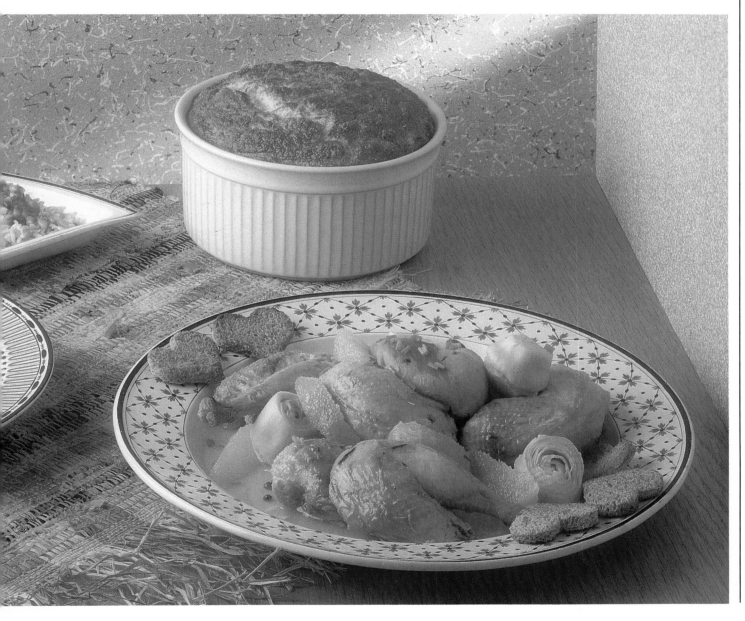

CLOCKWISE FROM LEFT Curried vegetables with brown rice; Salmon and cucumber soufflé; Pheasant with green peppercorns

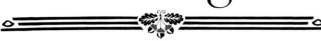

OCTOBER

Puddings

Passion Fruit Fool

6 ripe passion fruit
150 ml (¼ pint) skimmed
  milk
2 teaspoons cornflour
2 tablespoons water
150 ml (¼ pint) plain
  unsweetened yogurt
1 tablespoon clear honey

PREPARATION TIME:
20 minutes, plus chilling
COOKING TIME:
5 minutes
CALORIES PER PORTION:
135 (560 kilojoules)

1. Halve the passion fruit
and scoop out the pulp into
a bowl; discard the skins.
2. Gently heat the
skimmed milk. Blend the
cornflour and water to a

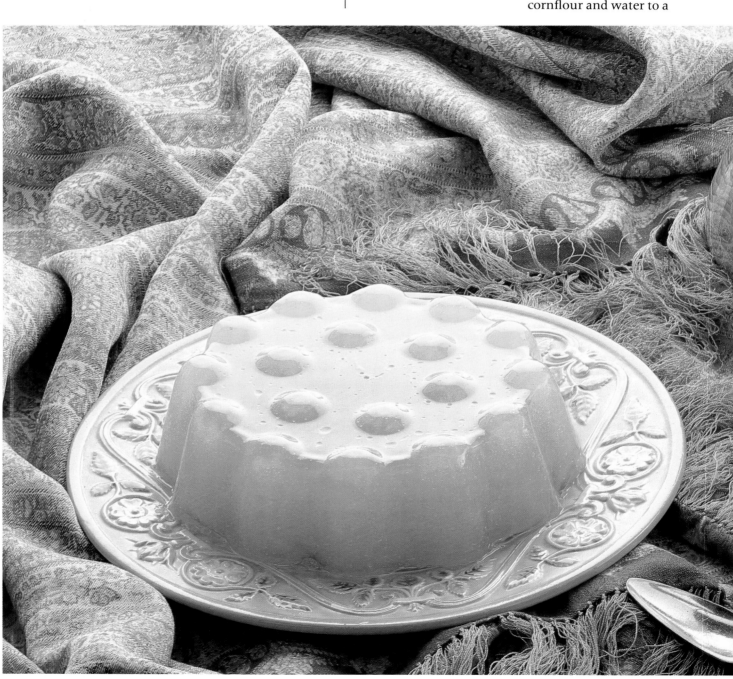

smooth paste; stir in the hot milk, return to the pan, and stir over the heat until the sauce has thickened. Remove from the heat and cool slightly.

3. Stir the yogurt and honey into the sauce and leave until quite cold.

4. Combine the sauce and passion fruit pulp. Spoon into serving dishes and chill for 3–4 hours.

Kiwi Fruit Salad

8 kiwi fruit
4 plump green grapes
8 plump black grapes
2 tablespoons dry white wine
2 tablespoons unsweetened orange juice

PREPARATION TIME:
25 minutes, plus chilling
CALORIES PER PORTION:
60 (250 kilojoules)

1. Peel the kiwi fruit and cut into thin slices; arrange these, overlapping, around the edges of 4 small plates.
2. Skin the green grapes and halve the black ones.
3. Arrange the black grapes in the centre of each plate; place a whole green grape in the centre of this.
4. Spoon the wine and the orange juice over and chill for 1 hour.

Quince Jelly

450 g (1 lb) quinces, roughly chopped
900 ml (1½ pints) water
½ lemon, thinly sliced
artificial sweetener, to taste
15 g (½ oz) powdered gelatine
175 g (6 oz) quince, sliced and poached, to decorate (optional)

PREPARATION TIME:
about 1 hour plus chilling
COOKING TIME:
1 hour
CALORIES PER PORTION:
55 (230 kilojoules)

1. Put the quinces into a pan with the water and sliced lemon; bring to the boil and simmer very gently for 1 hour.
2. Strain the liquid from the quinces through a muslin-lined sieve, allowing the juices to drip through naturally and slowly.
3. Make the quince juice up to 600 ml (1 pint) with water; add artificial sweetener to taste.
4. Put the gelatine and 3 tablespoons of the quince juice into a small bowl; stand in a pan of hot water and stir until the gelatine has dissolved.
5. Stir the dissolved gelatine into the remaining quince juice; pour into a lightly oiled 600 ml (1 pint) mould, and chill until set (about 3 hours).
6. Unmould the jelly on to a serving plate. Decorate with slices of poached quince if liked.

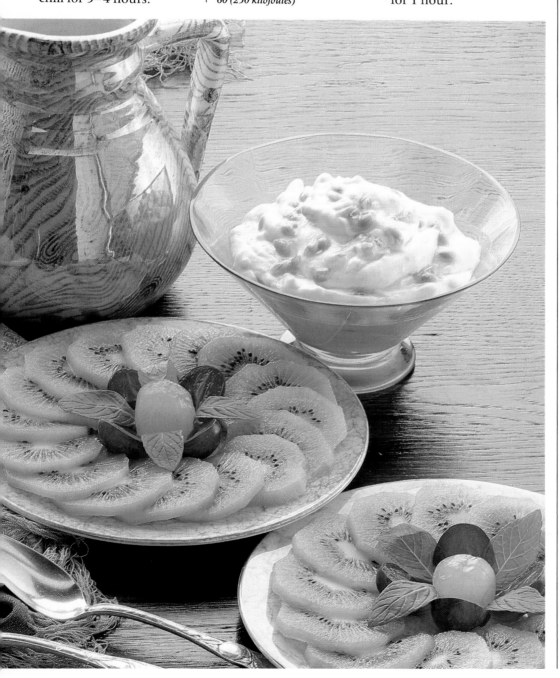

FROM THE LEFT Quince jelly; Kiwi fruit salad; Passion fruit fool

OCTOBER

Dinner Party for Six

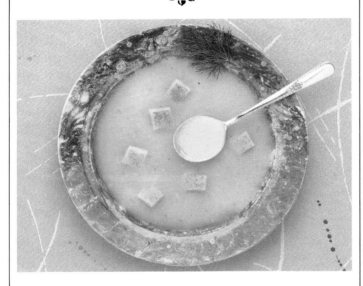

Jerusalem Artichoke Soup

500 g (1 lb 2 oz) Jerusalem
  artichokes, scraped clean
3 tablespoons lemon juice
1 tablespoon sunflower oil
900 ml (1½ pints)
  marrowbone or chicken stock
1 teaspoon dried dill
½ teaspoon sugar
salt
freshly ground black pepper
Lemon croûtons:
4 slices crustless bread
1 tablespoon lemon juice

PREPARATION TIME:
20 minutes
COOKING TIME:
45–50 minutes
OVEN TEMPERATURE:
200°C, 400°F, Gas Mark 6
CALORIES PER PORTION:
80 (340 kilojoules)

1. Chop the artichokes into small pieces, sprinkling them liberally with lemon juice as you work.
2. Heat the oil and add the artichokes, stir well. Cover and sweat over a gentle heat for 1–2 minutes. Pour on the stock, bring to the boil, cover and simmer for about 30 minutes.
3. Liquidize the artichokes, adding the dried dill and sugar, then push through a sieve and return to the pan. Reheat, and add salt and pepper to taste.
4. To make the lemon croûtons, brush both sides of the slices of bread with lemon juice and toast until lightly coloured on both sides. Cut into cubes.
5. Serve the soup, garnished with croûtons.

Poached Salmon Steaks with Hot Basil Sauce

1 large bunch fresh basil
4 celery sticks, chopped
1 carrot, peeled and chopped
1 small courgette, chopped
1 small onion, peeled and
  chopped
6 salmon steaks, about 100 g
  (4 oz) each and 2.5 cm
  (1 inch) thick
85 ml (3 fl oz) white wine
120 ml (4 fl oz) water
salt
freshly ground black pepper
1 teaspoon lemon juice
15 g (½ oz) unsalted butter

PREPARATION TIME:
15 minutes
COOKING TIME:
20–30 minutes
CALORIES PER PORTION:
260 (1090 kilojoules)

1. Strip the leaves off half the basil and set aside.
2. Spread all the chopped vegetables over the bottom of a large flameproof dish or pan with a lid, bed the salmon steaks in the vegetables and cover them with the remaining basil.
3. Pour over the wine and water and add salt and pepper to taste. Bring to the boil, cover and simmer for about 10 minutes. Transfer the salmon to a warmed serving dish.
4. Bring the poaching liquid and vegetables back to the boil and simmer for 5 minutes. Strain into a liquidizer and add the cooked and uncooked basil. Blend to a purée and return to a saucepan.
5. Bring the purée to the boil and reduce by half, until thickened.
6. Remove the pan from the heat, add the lemon juice and stir in the butter. Pour the sauce over the salmon steaks and serve.

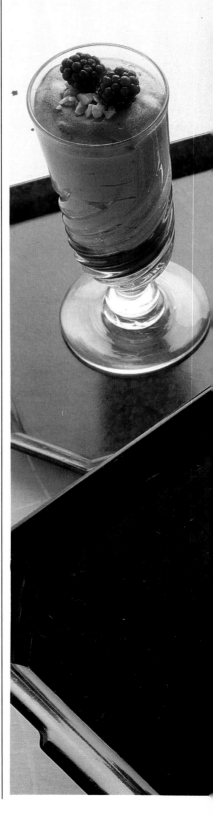

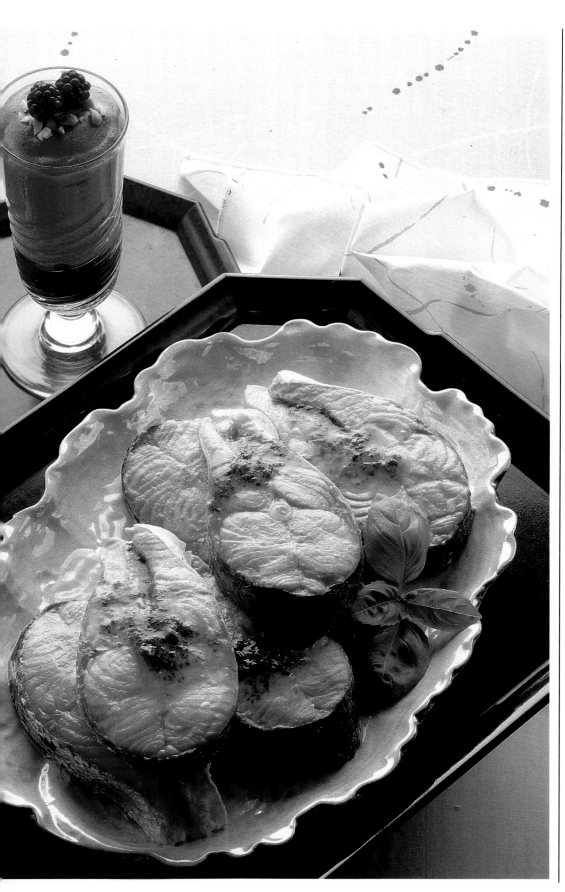

Blackberry Surprise

450 g (1 lb) blackberries
3 teaspoons clear honey
1 tablespoon lemon juice
1 sachet powdered gelatine
175 g (6 oz) plain
  unsweetened yogurt
4 Petit Suisse cheeses
2 egg whites
4 tablespoons port
1 tablespoon hazelnuts
2 slivers lemon rind, chopped

PREPARATION TIME:
20 minutes, plus cooling and chilling
COOKING TIME:
10–15 minutes
CALORIES PER PORTION:
165 (710 kilojoules)

1. Place half the blackberries in a thick-bottomed saucepan over a gentle heat and stir until softened. Stir in 2 teaspoons of honey.
2. Remove from the heat, add the lemon juice and sprinkle in the gelatine, stirring well to dissolve. Push through a sieve then leave the mixture to cool and thicken.
3. Combine the yogurt and Petit Suisse cheeses and stir in the cooled blackberry purée.
4. Whip the egg whites until stiff and fold in.
5. Reserve a few blackberries for decoration. Divide the remainder between 6 tall wineglasses and pour 1 tablespoon of port into each. Top up with mousse mixture and chill.
6. Just before serving, dry-fry the hazelnuts with the lemon rind. When evenly coloured chop them and sprinkle a little over each glass. Decorate with the remaining berries and honey.

OPPOSITE PAGE Jerusalem artichoke soup LEFT Poached salmon steaks with hot basil sauce; Blackberry surprise

NOVEMBER

Guy Fawkes Bonfire Party for Ten

If you had a cast-iron cauldron and tripod you could cook this gulyas (pronounced ghoulash) over the bonfire like the roaming Hungarian vagabonds of the past. As it is, it is less complicated to prepare it in the kitchen. The apples will cook in the hot ashes of the fire instead.

Pizza Mushrooms

1 dessertspoon olive oil
2 garlic cloves, peeled and
  quartered
1 teaspoon freshly ground
  coriander
12 green peppercorns
coarsely ground black pepper
salt
5 ripe medium tomatoes
  peeled, seeded and chopped
1 small can anchovy fillets,
  drained and chopped
20 open mushrooms about
  5 cm (2 inches) in diameter
75 g (3 oz) Edam cheese,
  grated
75 g (3 oz) fresh brown
  breadcrumbs
20 capers

PREPARATION TIME:
30 minutes
COOKING TIME:
7–10 minutes
CALORIES PER PORTION:
70 (295 kilojoules)

These are mini pizzas, using mushroom bases instead of bread, and can be served warm or cold and eaten with fingers around the bonfire.

1. Heat the oil and fry the garlic with the coriander, green peppercorns, black pepper and salt until golden.
2. Add the tomatoes and cook until soft. Add one-quarter of the anchovies, stir, remove from the heat and cool slightly.
3. Cut the stalks off the mushrooms level with the flesh. Wipe them clean, but do not wash them.
4. Mix the cheese and breadcrumbs together.
5. Spread the tomato mixture inside each mushroom. Place a caper and a piece of anchovy on each one and top with the breadcrumbs. Place under a preheated medium hot grill until crisp and sizzling.

Gulyas

25 g (1 oz) lard
2 large onions, peeled and
  finely chopped
1½ tablespoons sweet paprika
1.25 g (2¾ lb) flank steak,
  cut into 2.5 cm (1 inch) cubes
750 g (1½ lb) potatoes
1 teaspoon caraway seeds
2 tablespoons tomato purée
2.25 litres (4 pints)
  marrowbone or chicken stock
3 green peppers, seeded and
  sliced
salt
freshly ground black pepper

PREPARATION TIME:
15–18 minutes
COOKING TIME:
2–2½ hours
CALORIES PER PORTION:
255 (1065 kilojoules)

This is a substantial Hungarian soup. Csipetke (see next recipe) are essential for a genuine gulyas.

1. Heat the lard and fry the onions until well coloured. Remove from the heat and add the paprika.
2. Stir well and add the beef, one of the potatoes peeled and grated, and the caraway seeds. Stir and return to the heat, cover and simmer for 10–15 minutes, stirring from time to time.
3. Add the tomato purée and a cupful of the stock. Cover and simmer until the meat is nearly done. Add the remaining stock.
4. Peel and cube the remaining potatoes and add them with the green peppers as soon as the soup has come to the boil. Cook until the potatoes are done and the meat is tender. Add salt and pepper to taste.
5. Add the Csipetke (see next recipe) 10 minutes before serving and boil gently.

Csipetke

175 g (6 oz) plain flour
1 egg (size 1), lightly beaten
pinch of salt

PREPARATION TIME:
15–20 minutes
COOKING TIME:
10 minutes
CALORIES PER PORTION:
70 (295 kilojoules)

1. Sieve the flour on to a board, make a well in the centre and add the egg and the salt. With your hands work the mixture into a stiff dough. (If this proves to be impossible, add a

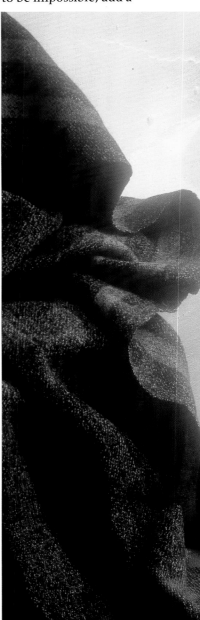

drop or two of water.)
2. Flatten the dough between the palms of your hands. Pinch off small pieces the size of kidney beans and add them to the slow boiling Gulyas 10 minutes before serving.

FROM THE TOP Pizza mushrooms; Gulyas with Csipetke; Bonfire cooked apples

Bonfire Cooked Apples

10 cooking apples, cored
100 g (4 oz) hazelnuts, toasted and ground
100 g (4 oz) seedless raisins, soaked in brandy for 1 hour
10 cloves
10 teaspoons unsweetened orange juice

PREPARATION TIME:
30 minutes, plus soaking
COOKING TIME:
30–40 minutes
CALORIES PER PORTION:
70 (295 kilojoules)

Just hand the foil balls to your guests and get them to put them in the glowing embers of the bonfire for about 10 minutes to heat through.

1. Make a series of little shallow slits in the skin of the apples, from top to bottom all the way around.
2. Mix together the hazelnuts and raisins and push them into the centre of each apple, adding a clove to each one.
3. Cut 10 pieces of foil, large enough when doubled to wrap each apple completely, allowing enough overlap to twist the corners at the top to form a handle. Double each piece, brush lightly with oil, lay an apple on each, pour over the orange juice and wrap.
4. Steam the foil-wrapped apples for 20–30 minutes over gently boiling water, but do not let them become too soft. Set aside until ready to finish the cooking.
5. Ten minutes before serving, put the apple parcels into the embers of the fire.

Menu continues over page

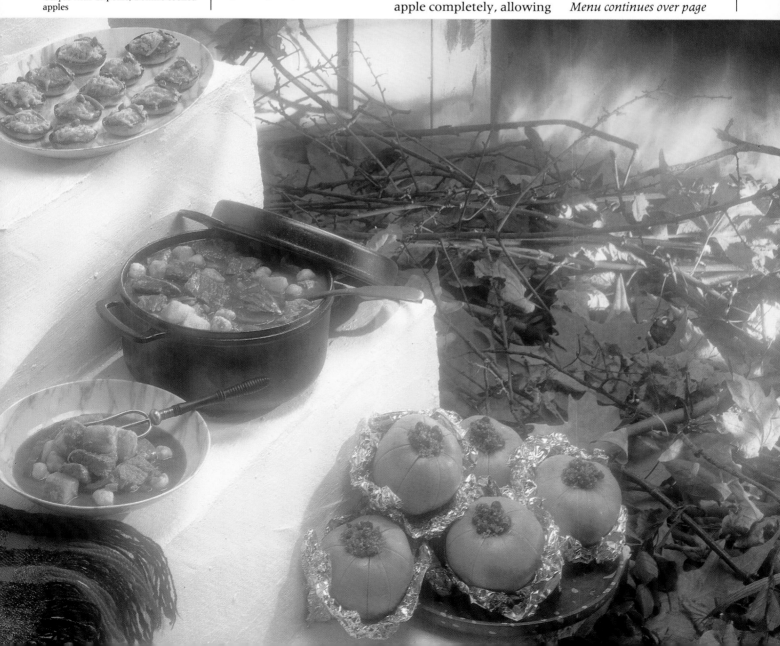

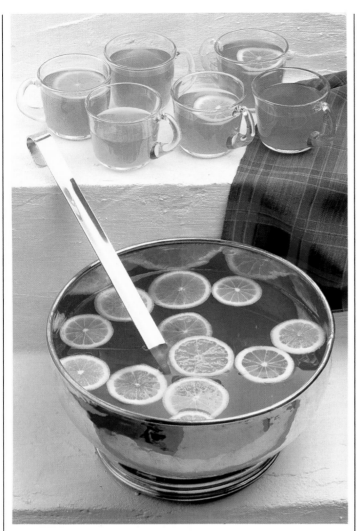

Tea, Rum and Orange Punch

10 medium oranges
1.75 litres (3 pints) hot tea, not too strong
2 lemons
1 cinnamon stick
250 ml (8 fl oz) dark rum
artificial sweetener, to taste

PREPARATION TIME:
20 minutes
COOKING TIME:
10 minutes
CALORIES PER PORTION:
55 (230 kilojoules)

This punch is best served warmed or hot for chilly nights, but it is also delicious iced.

1. Peel a very thin layer of skin off one of the oranges and steep it in the freshly made hot tea.
2. Squeeze the juice out of all the fruit except one half orange and one half lemon. Strain both juices and heat gently with the cinnamon stick.
3. Slice the half orange and half lemon as thinly as possible, soak the slices in the rum.
4. When the orange and lemon juice reaches boiling point stir it into the tea, add the rum with the fruit slices. Taste, and stir in artificial sweetener to taste. Remove the rind and cinnamon stick before serving.

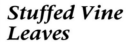

NOVEMBER

Hors d'oeuvres and Light Meals

Stuffed Vine Leaves

225 g (8 oz) preserved vine leaves, drained
175 g (6 oz) brown rice
1 small onion, peeled and finely chopped
2 tablespoons finely chopped fresh parsley
2 tablespoons finely chopped fresh mint
generous pinch of ground cinnamon
generous pinch of mixed spice
2 garlic cloves, peeled and crushed
50 g (2 oz) pine kernels, chopped
50 g (2 oz) currants
finely grated rind of ½ lemon
salt
freshly ground black pepper
250 ml (8 fl oz) water
12 black olives, to garnish

PREPARATION TIME:
45 minutes, plus cooling
COOKING TIME:
1½ hours
CALORIES PER PORTION:
240 (1010 kilojoules)

---

1. Put the vine leaves into a bowl and cover with boiling water. Agitate the leaves gently so that they separate.
2. Remove the leaves and drain them separately on paper towels.
3. Soak the brown rice in boiling water for 2–3 minutes, then rinse under cold water and drain well.
4. Mix the rice with the chopped onion, parsley, mint, cinnamon, mixed spice, garlic, pine kernels, currants, lemon rind and salt and pepper to taste.
5. Use a few damaged or mis-shapen leaves to line the base and sides of a large frying pan; reserve 4–6 perfect leaves for serving.
6. Divide the spiced rice mixture among the remaining leaves, placing it towards the stalk end of each leaf; fold in the edges and roll up the leaves, envelope fashion, so that the filling is completely enclosed. Pack the stuffed leaves closely together in the lined pan. Pour over the water.
7. Cover the pan with a tightly fitting lid, and simmer very gently for 1½ hours; top up with more water if the liquid evaporates too much during cooking.
8. Allow to cool in the pan. Place a perfect vine leaf on each serving plate, and arrange 5–6 stuffed leaves on top. Garnish each portion with a few black olives and serve.

ABOVE Tea, rum and orange punch
RIGHT, CLOCKWISE FROM TOP
Mushroom and parsley soup; Chick pea purée with vegetable sticks; Stuffed vine leaves

Chick Pea Purée with Vegetable Sticks

175 g (6 oz) chick peas, soaked
  overnight
1 teaspoon salt
1 bay leaf
small bunch of fresh mint
4 tablespoons lemon juice
2 large garlic cloves, peeled
  and crushed
1 tablespoon olive oil
4 tablespoons plain
  unsweetened yogurt
freshly ground black pepper
pinch of paprika
2–3 tablespoons warm water
To serve:
a selection of fresh vegetable
  sticks such as red and green
  peppers, celery, cucumber,
  carrots or French beans, plus
  trimmed radishes and
  broccoli florets

PREPARATION TIME:
10 minutes
COOKING TIME:
about 1 hour
CALORIES PER PORTION:
195 (815 kilojoules)

1. Drain the chick peas and
put them into a pan with
the salt, bay leaf and mint;
add sufficient water to
cover and simmer for 1
hour until tender. Drain and
remove bay leaf and mint.
2. Put the chick peas into
the liquidizer with the
lemon juice and garlic.
Blend until smooth,
gradually adding the olive
oil and yogurt. Add pepper
to taste, the paprika, and a
little warm water to adjust
consistency.
3. Serve with a selection of
prepared vegetables.

Mushroom and Parsley Soup

1 small onion, peeled and
  finely chopped
225 g (8 oz) button
  mushrooms, chopped
300 ml (½ pint) chicken stock
300 ml (½ pint) skimmed
  milk
3 tablespoons chopped fresh
  parsley
1 garlic clove, peeled and
  crushed
salt
freshly ground black pepper
3 tablespoons dry sherry
4 button mushrooms, thinly
  sliced, to garnish

PREPARATION TIME:
8–10 minutes
COOKING TIME:
about 15 minutes
CALORIES PER PORTION:
60 (250 kilojoules)

1. Put the chopped onion,
mushrooms, chicken stock,
milk, parsley and garlic into
a pan. Bring to the boil and
simmer for 10 minutes.
2. Blend the soup in the
liquidizer until smooth.
3. Put the soup into a
saucepan and add salt and
pepper to taste and the
sherry; heat through.
4. Serve the soup
garnished with sliced
mushrooms.

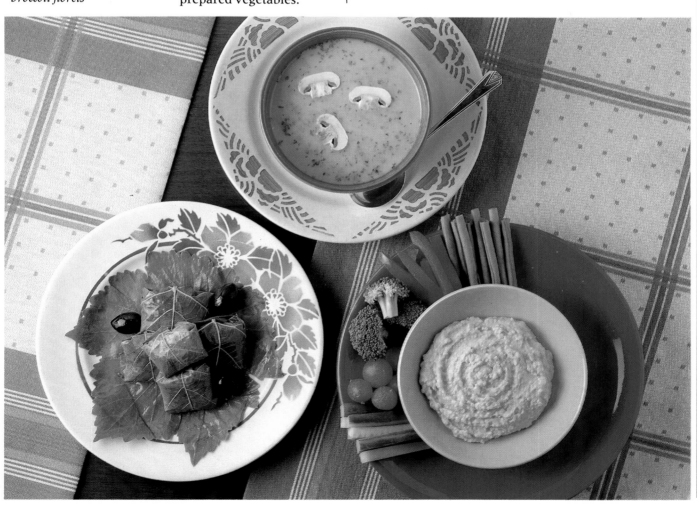

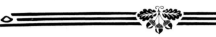

NOVEMBER

Main Courses

Dhal with Two Sauces

225 g (8 oz) green lentils, soaked overnight
1 small onion, peeled and finely chopped
thin slice of ginger root, finely chopped
2 fresh green chillies, chopped
2 bay leaves
2 garlic cloves, peeled and crushed
salt
freshly ground black pepper
sprigs of fresh coriander, to garnish

Tomato sauce:
1 small onion, peeled and finely chopped
1 tablespoon olive oil
450 g (1 lb) fresh tomatoes, skinned, seeded and chopped
1 garlic clove, peeled and crushed
1 tablespoon chopped fresh basil
4 tablespoons red wine

Avocado sauce:
3 spring onions, finely chopped
1 tablespoon olive oil
1 medium avocado, peeled, stoned and chopped
200 ml (1/3 pint) chicken stock
3 drops Tabasco sauce
2 tablespoons chopped fresh parsley
1 tablespoon lemon juice
grated rind of 1/2 lemon

PREPARATION TIME:
25 minutes
COOKING TIME:
1 hour 10 minutes
CALORIES PER PORTION:
250 (1050 kilojoules)

1. Drain the lentils and put into a large pan with the onion, ginger, chillies, bay leaves, garlic and salt and pepper to taste; add sufficient water to cover. Bring to the boil and simmer for about 1 hour, until the lentils are tender.
2. For the Tomato sauce, fry the onion gently in the olive oil for 3 minutes. Add the tomatoes, garlic, basil, wine and salt and pepper to taste; simmer gently for 8–10 minutes.
3. For the Avocado sauce, fry the spring onions gently in the olive oil for 3 minutes; add the chopped avocado, chicken stock, Tabasco, parsley, lemon juice, lemon rind and salt and pepper to taste; simmer gently for 5 minutes.
4. Spoon the cooked lentils into 2 mounds on 4 plates; spoon a different warm sauce over each one.
5. Garnish with sprigs of coriander and serve with a mixed salad.

Wild Duck with Satsuma Sauce

5 satsumas
1 small onion, peeled and finely chopped
4 tablespoons orange juice
2 tablespoons dry Vermouth
200 ml (1/3 pint) chicken stock
salt
freshly ground black pepper
2 wild ducks
4 sprigs fresh marjoram
4 rashers streaky bacon
4 tablespoons melted butter

PREPARATION TIME:
20–25 minutes
COOKING TIME:
1 hour 10 minutes
OVEN TEMPERATURE:
190°C, 375°F, Gas Mark 5
CALORIES PER PORTION:
350 (1470 kilojoules)

1. Peel the satsumas; separate the segments and remove all the pith.
2. Put the satsuma segments into a pan with the chopped onion, orange juice, Vermouth, stock and salt and pepper to taste; simmer gently for 5 minutes. Blend in the liquidizer until smooth.
3. Sprinkle the ducks inside and out with salt and pepper; put two sprigs of marjoram inside each bird. Stand them in a roasting tin, lay the bacon on the top and spoon over the melted butter.
4. Cover the ducks with foil and roast in a preheated oven for 45 minutes. Remove the foil and baste the ducks; return to the oven, uncovered, for about 15 minutes until just tender, but take care not to overcook.
5. Cut off the leg joints neatly; carve the breasts into thin slices.
6. Heat the satsuma sauce through gently. Serve the wild duck with the sauce spooned over the top.

Trout Fillets with Jerusalem Artichoke Purée

450 g (1 lb) Jerusalem artichokes, peeled
3–4 tablespoons lemon juice
2–3 tablespoons skimmed milk
salt
freshly ground black pepper
4 tablespoons dry white wine
4 medium trout, filleted into 2
175 g (6 oz) green grapes, skinned, halved and seeded
2 tablespoons finely chopped fresh parsley, to garnish

PREPARATION TIME:
15 minutes
COOKING TIME:
about 50 minutes
OVEN TEMPERATURE:
180°C, 350°C, Gas Mark 4
CALORIES PER PORTION:
390 (1640 kilojoules)

1. Cook the artichokes in boiling salted water for 15 minutes until tender. Drain.
2. Mash the artichokes to a purée with 1–2 tablespoons lemon juice, 2–3 tablespoons skimmed milk and salt and pepper to taste.
3. Combine 2 tablespoons lemon juice and the wine in a frying pan and poach the trout fillets for 6 minutes. Add halved grapes to the pan and cook for 1 minute.
4. Arrange on a serving dish and sprinkle with chopped parsley.
5. Serve with the hot Jerusalem artichoke purée.

FROM THE TOP Dhal with two sauces; Wild duck with satsuma sauce; Trout fillets with Jerusalem artichoke purée

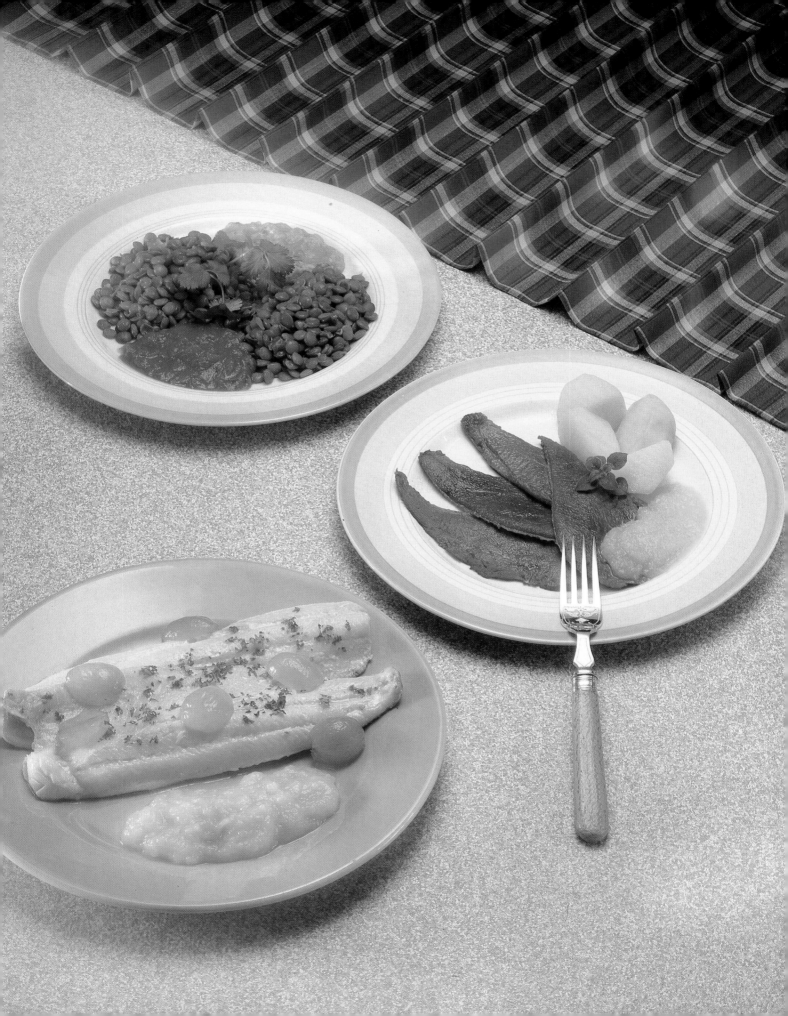

NOVEMBER

Puddings

Pineapple and Yogurt Cream

225 g (8 oz) canned pineapple in natural juice (drained weight), chopped
1 tablespoon clear honey
1 teaspoon grated lemon rind
1 egg yolk
300 ml (½ pint) plain unsweetened yogurt
3 teaspoons powdered gelatine
2 tablespoons water

To serve:
4 thin slices fresh pineapple
sprigs of fresh mint

PREPARATION TIME:
20 minutes, plus chilling
CALORIES PER PORTION:
120 (500 kilojoules)

1. Put the chopped pineapple, honey, lemon rind and egg yolk into the liquidizer; blend until smooth.
2. Mix the pineapple purée with the yogurt.
3. Put the gelatine and water in a small bowl standing in a pan of hot water and stir until dissolved. Mix into the pineapple mixture. Pour into 4 lightly greased 150 ml (¼ pint) dariole moulds and chill until set.
4. Place a slice of pineapple on 4 individual plates and carefully unmould a pineapple cream on to each one.
5. Decorate with sprigs of fresh mint and serve immediately.

Porcupine Pears

4 ripe pears
2 tablespoons lemon juice
20 split almonds, lightly toasted
200 ml (⅓ pint) low calorie ginger ale
1 tablespoon clear honey

PREPARATION TIME:
15–20 minutes
COOKING TIME:
2 minutes
CALORIES PER PORTION:
155 (650 kilojoules)

1. Peel the pears, leaving the stalks intact; carefully hollow out the core from the base of each pear. Brush all over with lemon juice.
2. Stud each pear with 10 pieces of split almond and sit each one on a small serving plate.
3. Heat the ginger ale with the honey; allow to cool slightly.
4. Spoon the ginger glaze over the pears while it is still warm. Serve immediately.

CLOCKWISE FROM LEFT Grapefruit sorbet; Porcupine pears; Pineapple and yogurt cream

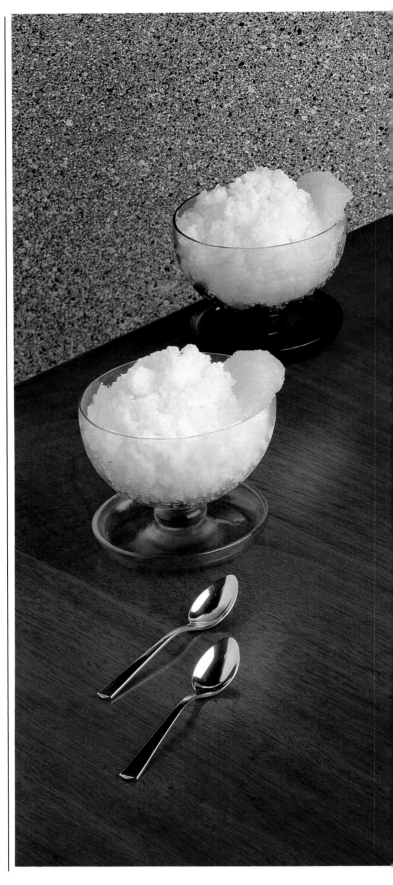

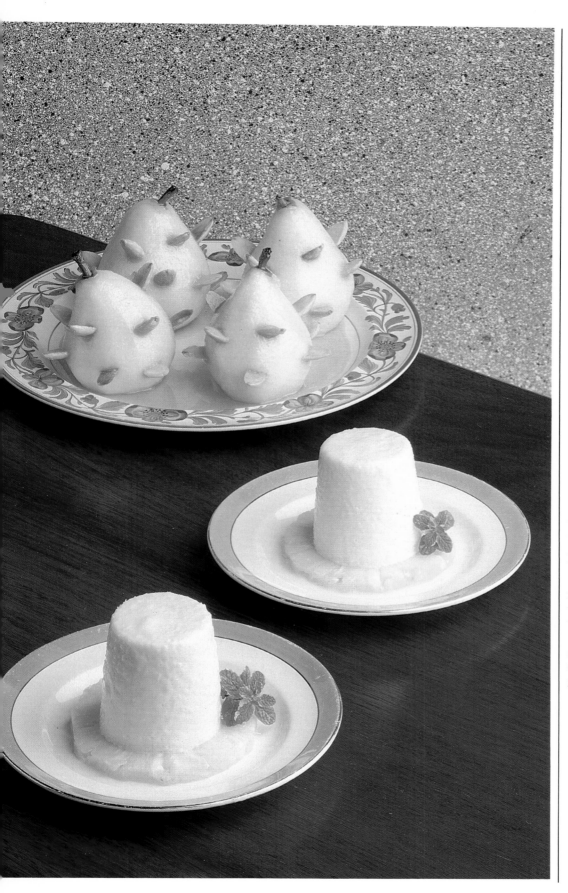

Grapefruit Sorbet

2 grapefruit
450 ml (¾ pint) water
artificial sweetener, to taste
3 tablespoons plain
  unsweetened yogurt
2 egg whites
peeled grapefruit segments, to
  decorate

PREPARATION TIME:
20–25 minutes, plus freezing
COOKING TIME:
about 10 minutes
CALORIES PER PORTION:
85 (355 kilojoules)

1. Thinly pare the rind from the grapefruit; cut the fruit in half and squeeze out the juice.
2. Put the pared grapefruit rind and the water into a pan; simmer gently for 8–10 minutes. Strain into a bowl and add the grapefruit juice and sweetener to taste.
3. Pour the grapefruit liquid into a shallow container and freeze until 'slushy' around the edges. Turn into a bowl and beat to break up the ice crystals.
4. Mix in the yogurt. Whisk the egg whites until stiff but not dry and fold into the grapefruit and yogurt mixture. Return to the freezer until firm.
5. Scoop the sorbet into stemmed glasses and decorate with peeled grapefruit segments.

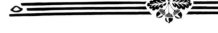

NOVEMBER

Dinner Party for Six

Vegetable Pâté

250 g (9 oz) chicken meat
1 small onion, peeled
1 small leek
2 celery sticks
200 g (7 oz) trimmed spinach
2 garlic cloves, chopped
1 tablespoon chopped mixed
 rosemary, thyme and parsley
1 egg, plus 1 egg white
1 tablespoon brandy
freshly ground black pepper
3 teaspoons Worcestershire
 sauce
150 ml (¼ pint) plain
 unsweetened yogurt

PREPARATION TIME:
15–20 minutes, plus chilling
COOKING TIME:
about 1¼ hours
OVEN TEMPERATURE:
190°C, 375°F, Gas Mark 5
CALORIES PER PORTION:
210 (880 kilojoules)

1. Mince the chicken,
onion, leek and celery
together with the spinach.
Add the garlic and herbs.
2. Lightly beat the egg with
the egg white and mix
with the brandy, pepper,
Worcestershire sauce and
yogurt. Stir into the
vegetable mixture.
3. Turn into a greased
terrine, cover with greased
foil and bake in a roasting
tin half filled with water
for about 1¼ hours.
4. Cool and refrigerate for
12 hours before serving.

Turkey Fillets with Piquant Prawn Sauce

3 red peppers, seeded and
 chopped
1 chilli, seeded and cut into 6
3 garlic cloves, peeled and
 chopped
3 tomatoes, skinned, seeded
 and chopped
1 aubergine, finely chopped
salt
freshly ground black pepper
6 turkey fillets, about
 175 g (6 oz) each
1 tablespoon olive oil
1 tablespoon vinegar
1 teaspoon anchovy essence
175 g (6 oz) peeled prawns

PREPARATION TIME:
20 minutes
COOKING TIME:
30–35 minutes
OVEN TEMPERATURE:
190–200°C, 375–400°F, Gas Mark
5–6
CALORIES PER PORTION:
250 (990 kilojoules)

1. Place all the chopped
vegetables in a bowl and
sprinkle with salt and
pepper, mix well.
2. Spread the mixture over
a sheet of foil large enough
to lay the fillets on side by
side. Place the meat on top
of the vegetables and paint
with a little of the oil.
Cover loosely with more
foil and seal completely.
Place on a baking tray in a
preheated oven (the oven
temperature depending on
the thickness of the fillets),
for 25–30 minutes.
Remove the fillets to a
warmed serving dish.
3. Heat the remaining oil in
a saucepan and push the
cooked vegetables through
a sieve on to it. Bring to the
boil and add the vinegar,
anchovy essence and
prawns, adjust the
seasoning and cook for
3–4 minutes. Spoon the
sauce over the fillets.

4. Serve with penne (pasta
quills) or plain rice that has
been mixed with diced
cucumber.

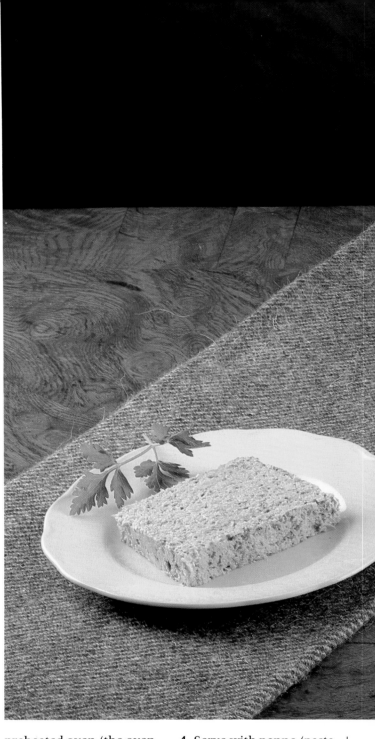

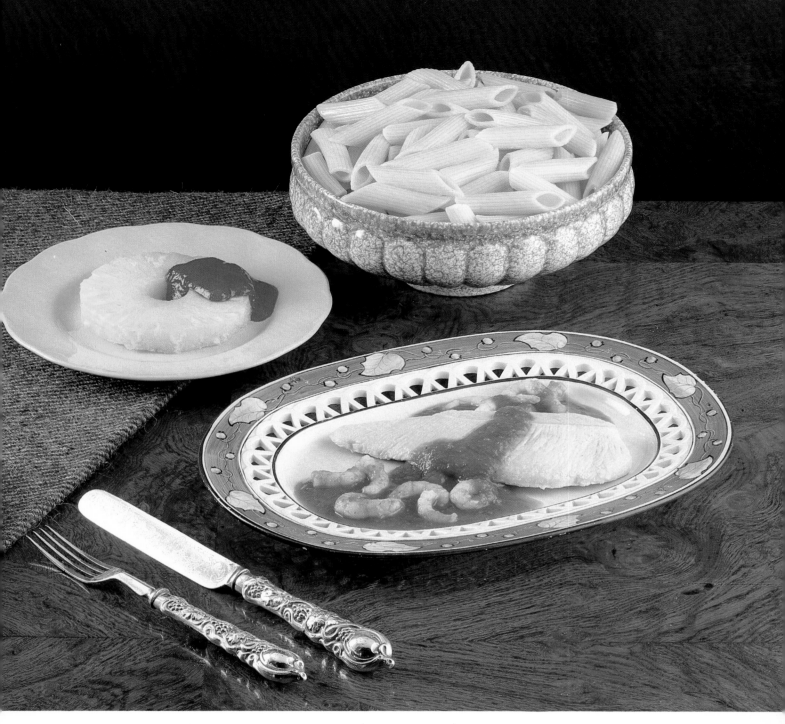

Pineapple under Cranberry

450 g (1 lb) cranberries
2 tablespoons cold water
2 teaspoons honey (optional)
6 pineapple slices, 2.5 cm
   (1 inch) thick, cored
6 tablespoons sweet cider

PREPARATION TIME:
10 minutes, plus cooling
COOKING TIME:
30 minutes
CALORIES PER PORTION:
80 (340 kilojoules)

Fresh cranberries are now in season, but if you cannot find them use frozen ones instead.

1. Put the cranberries in a saucepan with the cold water. Cover and cook gently until they are quite soft. Purée the cranberries by pushing them through a fine sieve, taste, and add the honey if necessary. Set aside in a warm place while you prepare the pineapple.
2. Cut the skins off the pineapple slices. Bring the cider to the boil in a large shallow pan, allow it to boil briskly for about 40 seconds then poach the slices until slightly softened but not mushy.

FROM THE LEFT Vegetable pâté; Pineapple under cranberry; Turkey fillets with piquant prawn sauce

(The length of time will depend on the ripeness of the fruit.)
3. Allow the pineapple slices to cool completely, then remove to a large shallow serving dish or individual plates and pour the slightly thickened cranberry purée over. Allow to cool and set before serving.

AUTUMN

Side Salads

Helios Salad

450 g (1 lb) carrots, coarsely
    shredded
25 g (1 oz) walnut pieces
120 ml (4 fl oz) unsweetened
    apple juice
120 ml (4 fl oz) plain
    unsweetened yogurt
½ teaspoon mixed spice
1 peach, stoned and roughly
    chopped

PREPARATION TIME:
10 minutes
CALORIES PER SERVING:
about 100 (420 kilojoules)

An unusual combination
of flavours, this autumn
salad is simply delicious.

1. Place the shredded
carrots in a serving dish.
2. Blend the walnuts with
half the apple juice in a
liquidizer, leaving some
walnut pieces intact to give
a nutty texture. Transfer to
a small bowl.
3. By hand, stir in the
remaining apple juice,
yogurt and mixed spice.
4. Stir the mixture and the
chopped peach into the
carrots and serve.

New Look Green Salad

350 g (12 oz) mixed salad
    leaves, washed and torn into
    pieces
175 g (6 oz) cucumber, grated
150 ml (¼ pint) cultured
    buttermilk or plain
    unsweetened yogurt
3 tablespoons chopped fresh
    mint, dill, basil or fennel
4 teaspoons grated Parmesan
    cheese
pinch of salt
1 clove garlic, peeled and
    crushed (optional)

PREPARATION TIME:
10 minutes
CALORIES PER SERVING:
about 90 (374 kilojoules)

Lettuce, watercress,
endive, chicory, young
dandelion leaves, spring
onions and mustard and
cress may all be used for
this salad.

1. Dry the salad leaves
thoroughly and arrange in
a salad bowl.
2. Blend all the other
ingredients together by
hand (a liquidizer or food
processor will make the
cucumber too mushy).
Pour into a jug.
3. To serve, let each guest
help themselves to the
salad leaves and hand the
sauce separately.

Egg and Mushroom Salad

3 tablespoons lemon juice
350 g (12 oz) flat or button
    mushrooms, washed but not
    peeled
2 teaspoons ground cumin or
    dried tarragon (optional)
1 crisp lettuce, cut into thick
    slices
150 ml (¼ pint) cultured
    buttermilk or plain
    unsweetened natural yogurt
2 hard-boiled eggs, finely
    chopped
freshly ground black pepper

PREPARATION TIME:
12 minutes, plus standing
CALORIES PER SERVING:
about 90 (370 kilojoules)

You can use the
mushroom stalks as well as
the caps in this recipe. The
lettuce slices make
miniature 'plates' which
quickly take on the
flavours of the salad.

1. Put the lemon juice in a
bowl and slice the
mushrooms thinly directly
into the lemon juice to
prevent discoloration. Add
the cumin or tarragon (if
using) and toss well. Drain,
reserving any juice.
2. Divide the lettuce slices
between 4 plates.
3. Spoon the mushrooms
on top, then mix the
lemon juice left in the bowl
with the buttermilk or
yogurt and the chopped
eggs. Spoon the mixture
over the mushrooms.
4. Sprinkle each salad
generously with black
pepper and leave to stand
for 15 minutes before
serving to allow the
flavours to blend.

Apple and Plum Salad

350 g (12 oz) apples, washed
2 tablespoons orange juice
225 g (8 oz) Victoria plums,
    washed, halved and stoned
225 g (8 oz) cottage cheese
50 g (2 oz) reduced fat hard
    cheese, grated
15 g (½ oz) flaked almonds
¼ teaspoon black pepper

PREPARATION TIME:
10 minutes
CALORIES PER SERVING:
about 170 (710 kilojoules)

Ideal for those who like
eating with their fingers,
this salad is served like a
dip, with the apple slices
arranged around a small
mound of cheese on each
person's plate.

1. Quarter and slice the
apples and toss
immediately in the orange
juice to prevent
discoloration.
2. Cut the plum halves into
quarters, then arrange
with the apple slices on 4
plates.
3. Put the soft and hard
cheeses in a bowl and
mash together with a fork.
Spoon a mound of the
cheese mixture on to each
plate.
4. Place the almonds under
a preheated grill and toast
for 2 minutes.
5. Sprinkle each mound of
cheese with pepper and
flaked almonds and serve.

CLOCKWISE FROM TOP RIGHT New
look green salad: Apple and plum
salad; Helios salad; Egg and mushroom
salad

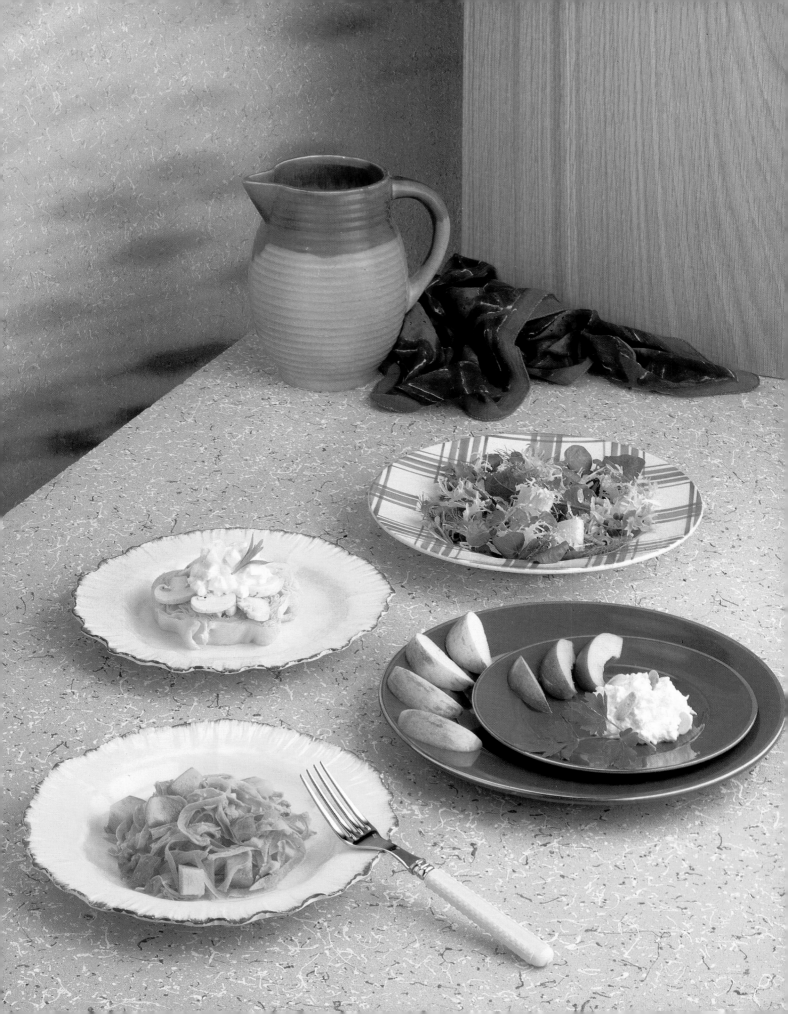

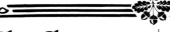

AUTUMN

Main Course Salads

Blue Cheese Pears

100 g (4 oz) Danish blue
 cheese
225 g (8 oz) cottage cheese or
 smooth low fat cheese
2 celery sticks, chopped
50 g (2 oz) hazelnuts, chopped
6 large pears
2 tablespoons lemon juice
salad burnet leaves, to
 garnish

PREPARATION TIME:
10 minutes
CALORIES PER SERVING:
about 320 (1325 kilojoules)

1. Mash the blue cheese,
soft cheese and celery
together.
2. Place the chopped nuts
in an ungreased heavy-
based frying pan over a
low heat and stir for 2–3
minutes until slightly
browned. Place in a bowl.
3. Peel and halve the pears
and scoop out the cores
with a teaspoon. Brush
immediately with the
lemon juice.
4. Fill the centres of the
pears with about half the
cheese mixture. Place 3,
cut side down, on 4 plates.
5. With the help of a
teaspoon, shape the
remaining cheese mixture
into 12 balls the size of
large marbles. Roll each
one in the bowl of nuts.
Place 3 on each plate.
6. Garnish each plate with
salad burnet and serve.

Julienne Chicken Salad

100 g (4 oz) eating apple
1 tablespoon lemon juice
450 g (1 lb) cooked chicken,
 cut into thin strips
100 g (4 oz) cucumber, cut
 into thick matchstick strips
100 g (4 oz) small turnips or
 chicory, cut into thick
 matchstick strips
100 g (4 oz) red pepper, cored
 seeded and cut into rings,
 each ring cut into 4
1 tablespoon mango chutney
100 g (4 oz) cottage cheese
2 teaspoons red wine vinegar
1 tablespoon sunflower oil
2 tablespoons chopped fresh
 parsley
To serve:
100 g (4 oz) wholemeal toast,
 cut into fingers

PREPARATION TIME:
15 minutes
CALORIES PER SERVING:
about 285 (1190 kilojoules)

1. Cut the apple into thick
matchstick strips and toss
in the lemon juice
immediately to avoid
discoloration.
2. Mix the apple with the
chicken, cucumber,
turnips or chicory and red
pepper in a serving bowl.
3. Blend the chutney,
cottage cheese, vinegar, oil
and parsley together in the
liquidizer.
4. Spoon the dressing over
the salad and serve with
the wholemeal toast.

Tabbouleh

175 g (6 oz) bulgar wheat
50 g (2 oz) roughly chopped
 fresh parsley
2 tablespoons chopped fresh
 mint
1 bunch spring onions,
 trimmed and finely chopped
2 cloves garlic, peeled and
 crushed (optional)
2 tablespoons lemon juice
1 tablespoon olive or
 sunflower oil
¼ teaspoon freshly ground
 black pepper
pinch of salt
100 g (4 oz) Cheshire cheese,
 cut into 1 cm (½ inch) cubes
8 green olives

PREPARATION TIME:
5 minutes, plus soaking
CALORIES PER SERVING:
about 300 (1255 kilojoules)

A traditional Lebanese
salad that's delightfully
easy to prepare. It should
contain almost as much
greenery as wheat.

1. Boil a kettle. Place the
wheat in a sieve sitting in a
large bowl which is about
the same depth as the
sieve.
2. Pour boiling water over
the wheat to cover. Leave
to absorb for 20 minutes,
adding a little more water
if the wheat appears dry.
3. Meanwhile, combine all
the remaining ingredients
except the cheese and
olives in a serving dish.
4. When the wheat is
tender, lift the sieve from
the bowl, pressing down
on the wheat to push out
any excess water. Transfer
to the serving dish and toss
to distribute the dressing
evenly.
5. Sprinkle the cubed
cheese and olives over and
serve.

Salade Niçoise

225 g (8 oz) potatoes, washed
 but not peeled
225 g (8 oz) French beans,
 trimmed and cut into 4 cm
 (1½ inch) lengths
225 g (8 oz) tomatoes, washed
 and cut into wedges
1 red or green pepper, cored,
 seeded and diced
1 mild onion, about 150 g
 (5 oz), peeled and finely
 chopped
1 × 200 g (7 oz) can tuna in
 brine, drained
2 hard-boiled eggs, quartered
8 black olives
Dressing:
1 tablespoon olive or
 sunflower oil (see below)
50 ml (2 fl oz) red wine
 vinegar
1 teaspoon tomato ketchup
2 teaspoons unrefined brown
 sugar
1 teaspoon chilli sauce
 (optional)
1 tablespoon water
1 clove garlic, peeled and
 crushed (optional)
pinch of dry mustard

PREPARATION TIME:
25 minutes
COOKING TIME:
about 25 minutes
CALORIES PER SERVING:
about 350 (1465 kilojoules)

Full of the tastes of the
Mediterranean, this salad
will benefit if first-pressing
'virgin' olive oil is used in
the dressing. This is the
highest quality olive oil
available, produced by
crushing the fresh cold
olives without heating or
other processing. It should
be a clear green colour and
have a distinctive aroma
which blends perfectly
with garlic. The authentic
Niçois version of this salad
does not include boiled
potato, but in this
slimmer's version cooked
potatoes and French beans
supply valuable fibre and
body.

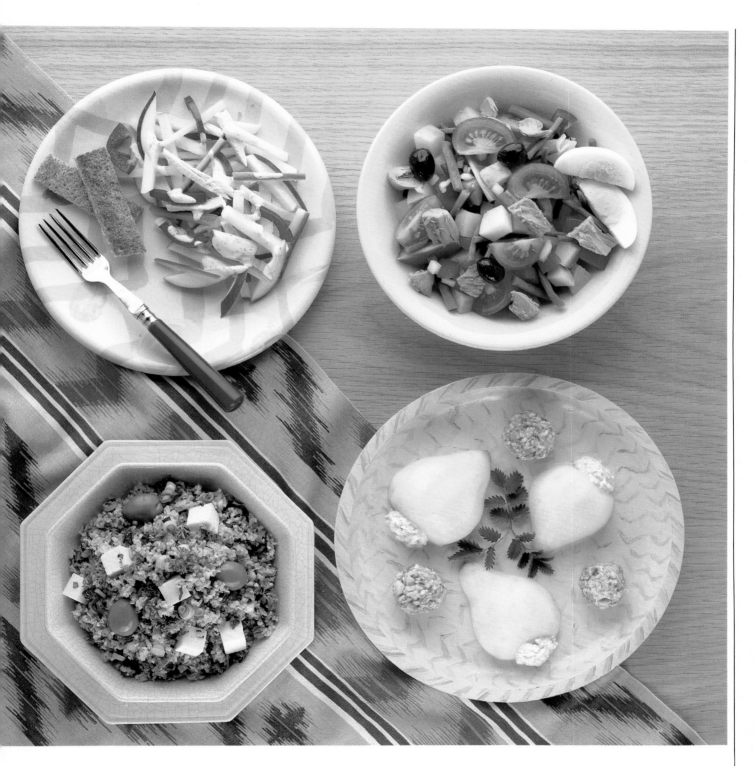

1. Boil or steam the potatoes until just tender – about 20 minutes. Drain and dice.
2. Blanch the beans by plunging them into a saucepan containing 1 cm (½ inch) depth of boiling water. Bring back to the boil, cover and simmer for 5 minutes. Drain.
3. Combine the potatoes, beans, tomatoes, pepper, onion and tuna in a serving dish.
4. Place all the dressing ingredients in a screw-topped jar and shake well. Pour over salad and toss well.
5. Arrange the egg quarters and olives on top and serve.

CLOCKWISE FROM TOP LEFT
Julienne chicken salad; Salade Niçoise; Blue cheese pears; Tabbouleh

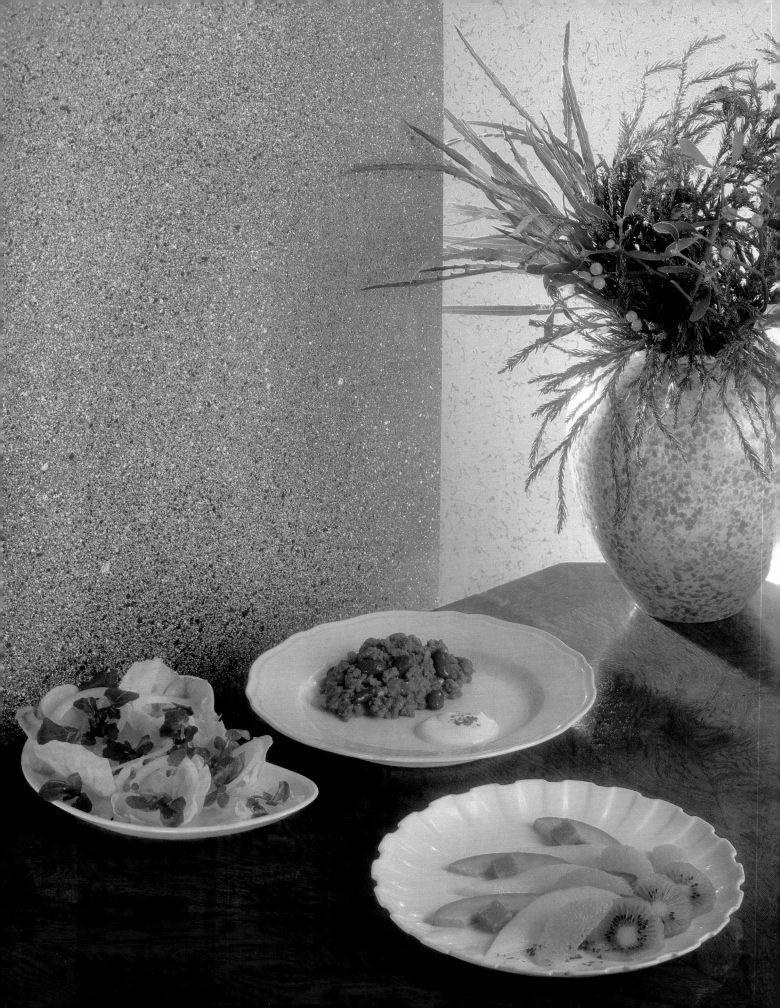

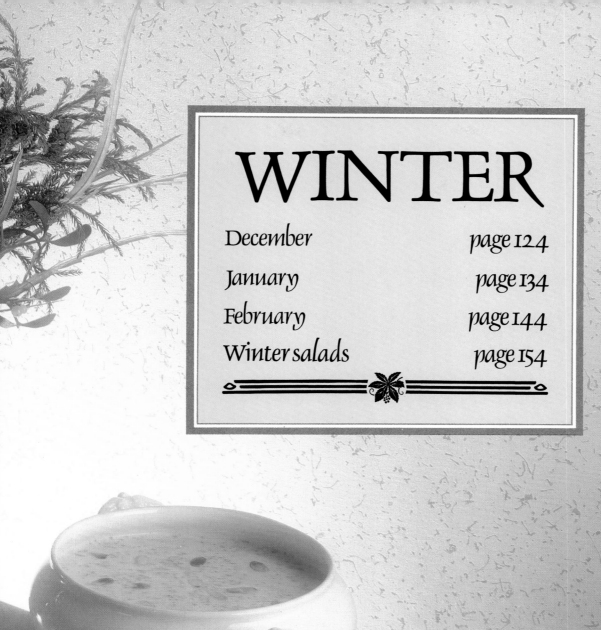

WINTER

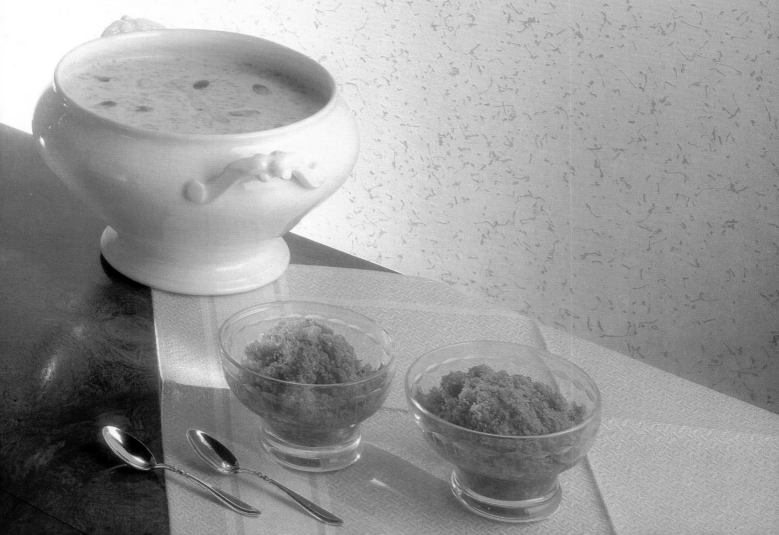

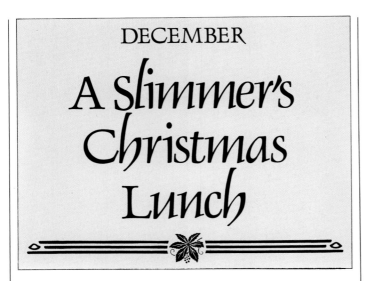

DECEMBER
A Slimmer's Christmas Lunch

This menu includes all the familiar flavours of Christmas but avoids the equally traditional high calorie count. Serves 8.

Turkey Parcels

8 turkey escalopes, about
*   150 g (5 oz) each*
300 ml (½ pint) white wine
300 ml (½ pint) turkey or
*   chicken stock*
Stuffing:
225 g (8 oz) courgettes, grated
75 g (3 oz) hazelnuts, toasted
*   and ground*
2 spring onions, trimmed and
*   finely chopped*
½ tablespoon lime juice
1 teaspoon grated lime rind
1 teaspoon clear honey
1 teaspoon grated fresh ginger
1 teaspoon fresh or dried
*   thyme*
coarsely ground black pepper

PREPARATION TIME:
40 minutes
COOKING TIME:
35–40 minutes
CALORIES PER PORTION:
270 (1110 kilojoules)

1. Holding the knife horizontally, cut a 5 cm (2 inch) slit in each escalope pushing the knife deep into the flesh to make a pocket. Make sure that you do not cut through the flesh.
2. Combine all the stuffing ingredients together in a mixing bowl, adding black pepper to taste.
3. Divide the stuffing between the escalopes, pushing the stuffing well into the pockets.
4. Combine the wine and stock. Pour into one or two large shallow pans and bring to the boil. Reduce to a very gentle simmer and poach the escalopes, stuffing side up, for 20–25 minutes, until cooked through.
5. Remove the escalopes with a slotted spoon and drain on paper towels. Transfer to a heated serving dish and keep warm.
6. Boil the poaching liquid fast until reduced to about 150 ml (¼ pint).
7. Spoon a little of the reduced cooking juices over each escalope and serve, accompanied by Gingered Brussels sprouts and potatoes or rice.

CLOCKWISE, FROM RIGHT Gingered Brussels sprouts; Turkey parcels; Apricot and apple whip; Carrot and sage soup

Carrot and Sage Soup

25 g (1 oz) butter
1 large onion, peeled and
*   finely chopped*
750 g (1½ lb) carrots, scraped
*   and finely sliced*
1.75 litres (3 pints) stock
salt
pepper
1 tablespoon chopped fresh
*   sage*
sprigs of fresh sage leaves
*   (optional), to garnish*

PREPARATION TIME:
15 minutes
COOKING TIME:
about 1 hour
CALORIES PER PORTION:
45 (185 kilojoules)

Fresh sage is often available during the winter months, but dried sage may be used instead. Soak it first in a tablespoon of warmed white wine.

1. Melt the butter in a large heavy-based pan and gently fry the onion until transparent, then add the carrots and stock. Season with salt and pepper.
2. Bring to the boil and simmer uncovered for about 30 minutes.
3. Liquidize the soup then return to the pan and add the chopped sage. Bring to the boil and simmer for another 15 minutes.
4. Serve, garnished with sage sprigs.

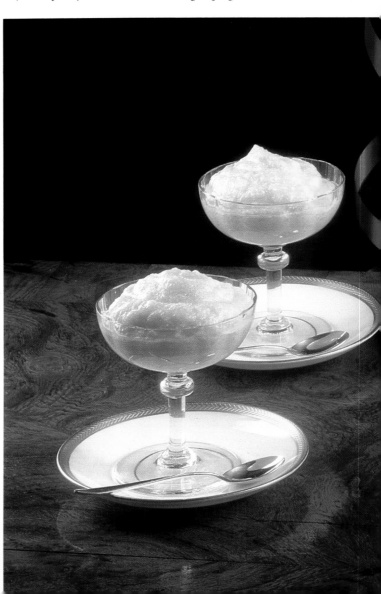

Gingered Brussels Sprouts

1.25 kg (2¾ lb) Brussels
  sprouts (see right)
2 tablespoons lemon juice
1 teaspoon finely grated fresh
  ginger or ½ teaspoon
  ground ginger
3–4 strips lemon rind

PREPARATION TIME:
10 minutes, plus standing
COOKING TIME:
8–10 minutes
CALORIES PER PORTION:
30 (125 kilojoules)

Prepare the sprouts by
trimming the ends and
removing any discoloured
outer leaves. Do not cut a
cross in the ends if you
want them to be slightly
crunchy.

1. Steam the sprouts for
8 minutes then pour the
water out of the pan under
the steamer and put the
sprouts into the hot pan to
dry out slightly.
2. Sprinkle the lemon juice
and ginger over, toss well
and add the strips of lemon
rind.
3. Cover and leave to stand
in a warm place for 5
minutes before serving.

Apricot and Apple Whip

225 g (8 oz) dried apricot
  halves
600 ml (1 pint) water
225 g (8 oz) sliced dessert
  apples
2 egg whites
½ teaspoon ground cinnamon
¼ teaspoon ground nutmeg

PREPARATION TIME:
20 minutes
COOKING TIME:
45 minutes
CALORIES PER PORTION:
65 (275 kilojoules)

1. Place the apricots in a
saucepan and add 450 ml
(¾ pint) of the water.

Bring to the boil, cover and
simmer until all the water
is absorbed and the fruit is
quite mushy. Cook the
apple slices in the
remaining water just until
soft.
2. Pass each fruit through a
sieve into separate bowls.
Beat the egg whites until
stiff and fold half into each
fruit purée, adding the
cinnamon to the apple and
the nutmeg to the apricots.
3. To serve, spoon a layer
of apricot purée into
individual glasses, then
spoon in a layer of apple.

Menu continues over page

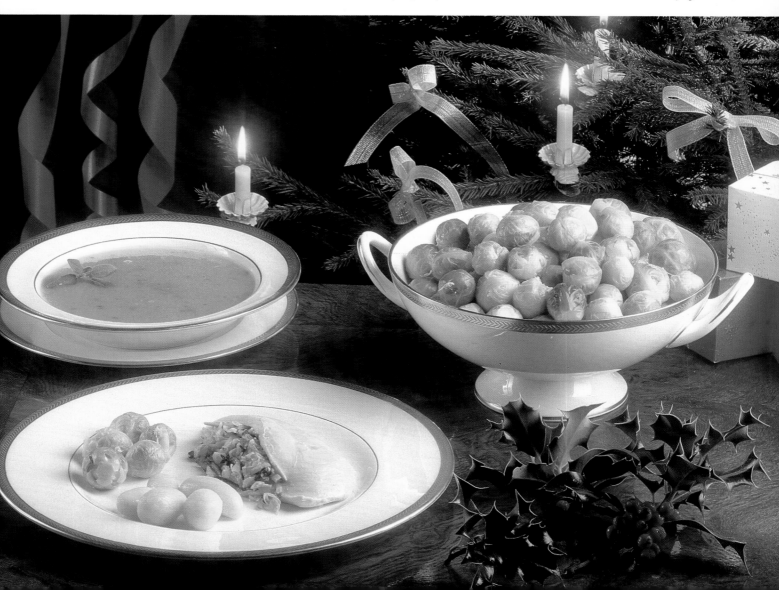

Christmas Carrot Cake

175 g (6 oz) sultanas
4 tablespoons whisky
250 ml (8 fl oz) corn oil
100 g (4 oz) molasses sugar
  (natural and unrefined)
3 eggs (size 1)
1 tablespoon cocoa
225 g (8 oz) plain 85%
  wholemeal flour
1 teaspoon cinnamon
½ teaspoon nutmeg
½ teaspoon allspice
½ teaspoon salt
1½ teaspoons baking powder
1½ teaspoons bicarbonate of
  soda
225 g (8 oz) carrots, finely
  grated
75 g (3 oz) walnuts, finely
  chopped
Icing:
50 g (2 oz) icing sugar
350 g (12 oz) low fat soft
  cheese
rind of ½ lemon, finely grated

PREPARATION TIME:
30 minutes, plus soaking
COOKING TIME:
1¼ hours
OVEN TEMPERATURE:
180°C, 350°F, Gas Mark 4
CALORIES PER SLICE
(MAKES 16 SLICES):
300 (1260 kilojoules)

This recipe is just as good as our traditional fruit cake but has significantly fewer Calories.

1. Soak the sultanas in the whisky for 1 hour or more.
2. Line a loose bottomed 20 cm (8 inch) cake tin with non-stick silicone, or greased and floured greaseproof paper.
3. Beat together the oil and sugar, adding the eggs one at a time. (At this stage the mixture looks very odd, but don't worry.)
4. Still beating, add the cocoa, flour, spices, salt, baking powder and bicarbonate of soda.
5. Mix in the carrots, the sultanas and the whisky, if it has not all been absorbed, and the nuts. Stir and tip the mixture into the cake tin.
6. Bake in a preheated oven for about 1¼ hours; a warmed skewer will come out clean when the cake is cooked. Allow the cake to cool in the tin.
7. Work the icing sugar into the soft cheese and add the lemon rind. When the cake is quite cold, spread the icing over it.

BELOW Christmas carrot cake

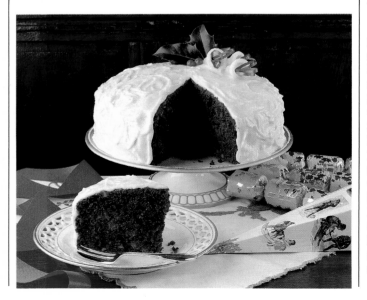

Hors d'oeuvres and Light Meals

Celery and Almond Soup

1 small onion, peeled and
  finely chopped
6 celery sticks, finely chopped
1 tablespoon coarsely chopped
  fresh parsley
1 teaspoon dill seed
50 g (2 oz) blanched almonds
300 ml (½ pint) chicken stock
300 ml (½ pint) skimmed
  milk
3 tablespoons plain
  unsweetened yogurt
1 egg yolk
1 tablespoon toasted flaked
  almonds, to garnish

PREPARATION TIME:
15 minutes
COOKING TIME:
15 minutes
CALORIES PER PORTION:
140 (590 kilojoules)

1. Put the onion, celery, parsley, dill seed, almonds, stock and milk into a pan; bring to the boil and simmer gently for about 12 minutes until the vegetables are tender.
2. Blend the soup in the liquidizer until smooth. Return to a clean saucepan. Beat the yogurt with the egg yolk and stir into the soup.
3. Reheat the soup gently; do not allow it to boil. Ladle into small bowls and sprinkle with the toasted almonds.

Avocado and Fruit Salad

4 tablespoons orange juice
1 tablespoon olive oil
salt
freshly ground black pepper
1 garlic clove, peeled and
  crushed
1 tablespoon chopped fresh
  mint
1 large avocado pear, peeled,
  halved, stoned and sliced
1 large orange, divided into
  segments
1 kiwi fruit, peeled and sliced
100 g (4 oz) melon, cut into
  thin slivers
75 g (3 oz) lean smoked ham,
  cut into small cubes
sprigs of fresh parsley, to
  garnish

PREPARATION TIME:
about 40 minutes
CALORIES PER PORTION:
110 (460 kilojoules)

1. To make the dressing, mix the orange juice with the olive oil, salt and pepper to taste, the garlic and chopped mint.
2. Arrange the sliced avocado decoratively on 4 small plates with the orange segments, kiwi fruit slices and slivers of melon; arrange the cubes of smoked ham on top.
3. Spoon the prepared dressing over the arranged fruits and garnish each plate with a sprig of parsley.

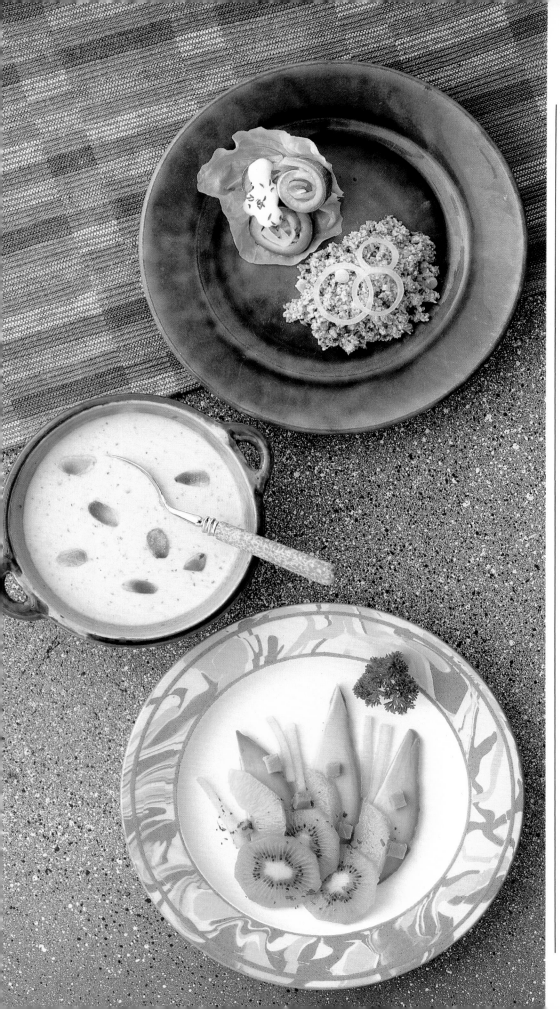

Herring and Cracked Wheat Salad

100 g (4 oz) bulgar (cracked
  wheat)
3 spring onions, finely
  chopped
1 garlic clove, peeled and
  finely chopped
3 tablespoons finely chopped
  parsley
salt
freshly ground black pepper
2 tablespoons lemon juice
1 tablespoon olive oil
4 rollmop herrings
4 centre lettuce leaves
3 tablespoons plain
  unsweetened yogurt
To garnish:
thin onion rings
caraway seeds

PREPARATION TIME:
20–25 minutes, plus soaking
CALORIES PER PORTION:
270 (1130 kilojoules)

1. Soak the bulgar in warm
water for 30 minutes;
squeeze out the excess
moisture and drain the
bulgar on a clean cloth.
2. Mix the prepared bulgar
in a bowl with the spring
onions, garlic, parsley, salt
and pepper to taste, lemon
juice and olive oil.
3. Cut each rollmop in half,
place on a lettuce leaf on a
small serving plate and
spoon over a little yogurt.
4. Spoon a pile of the
prepared bulgar next to the
herring, garnish with thin
onion rings and a
sprinkling of caraway seeds
and serve.

FROM THE TOP Herring and cracked
wheat salad; Celery and almond soup;
Avocado and fruit salad

DECEMBER

Main Courses

Soufflé Cheese Potatoes

4 medium potatoes, washed
20 g (¾ oz) butter
salt
freshly ground black pepper
100 g (4 oz) curd cheese
2 tablespoons grated
  Parmesan cheese
2 teaspoons French or
  wholegrain mustard
2 eggs, separated

PREPARATION TIME:
25 minutes
COOKING TIME:
about 1½ hours
OVEN TEMPERATURE:
190°C, 375°F, Gas Mark 5
CALORIES PER PORTION:
250 (1050 kilojoules)

1. Place the potatoes on a baking sheet and bake in a preheated oven for about 1¼ hours, until tender.
2. Cut a lengthways slice from the top of each potato; carefully scoop most of the centre potato into a bowl, leaving a shell.
3. Mix the centre potato with the butter, salt and pepper to taste, curd cheese, 1 tablespoon of Parmesan, the mustard and egg yolks.
4. Whisk the egg whites until stiff but not dry; fold lightly into the potato mixture. Spoon into the potato shells then sprinkle with the remaining cheese.
5. Return the potatoes to the oven for a further 15–20 minutes, until well risen, golden and puffed.
6. Serve immediately.

Veal Paupiettes

4 veal escalopes, flattened,
  about 150 g (5 oz) each
1 teaspoon grated lemon rind
1 small onion, chopped
freshly ground black pepper
1 tablespoon chopped sage
4 large lettuce leaves
20 g (¾ oz) butter
1 tablespoon olive oil
150 ml (¼ pint) white wine
150 ml (¼ pint) chicken stock
2 medium parsnips, peeled,
  chopped and cooked
2 tablespoons plain
  unsweetened yogurt
2 canned red pimentos
1 tablespoon chopped chives
salt

PREPARATION TIME:
20 minutes
COOKING TIME:
20–25 minutes
CALORIES PER PORTION:
300 (1260 kilojoules)

1. Sprinkle the escalopes with rind, onion, pepper and sage. Lay a lettuce leaf on top of each and roll up. Tie neatly.
2. Heat the butter and oil in a shallow pan; add the prepared veal paupiettes and cook until evenly coloured on all sides. Add the wine and chicken stock; cover and simmer until the veal is tender.
3. Meanwhile, blend the parsnips, yogurt and red pimentos in the liquidizer. Mix in the chives and season. Heat through in a double saucepan.
4. Spoon the purée on to a serving dish and arrange the paupiettes on top.

Sesame Turkey with Ginger and Lychees

450 g (1 lb) turkey fillets cut
  into thin strips
1 egg, beaten
3 tablespoons sesame seeds
3 tablespoons olive oil
1 small onion, peeled and
  finely chopped
1 garlic clove, peeled and
  finely chopped
slice of fresh ginger, 1 cm
  (½ inch) thick, finely
  chopped
2 tablespoons unsweetened
  pineapple juice
4 tablespoons chicken stock
12 fresh lychees, shelled
1 tablespoon lime juice
salt
freshly ground black pepper
julienne strips of spring
  onion, to garnish

PREPARATION TIME:
20–25 minutes
COOKING TIME:
20 minutes
CALORIES PER PORTION:
285 (1190 kilojoules)

1. Dip the strips of turkey into beaten egg, shaking off the excess, and coat lightly in sesame seeds.
2. Heat the olive oil in a large shallow pan; add the onion and garlic and fry for 2–3 minutes. Add the ginger and the strips of turkey and fry until the turkey is evenly coloured.
3. Pour over the pineapple juice and stock and simmer for 5 minutes, covered.
4. Add the lychees and lime juice and season to taste. Stir well then simmer, covered for a further 4–5 minutes.
5. Serve, garnished with spring onion strips on a bed of Chinese noodles.

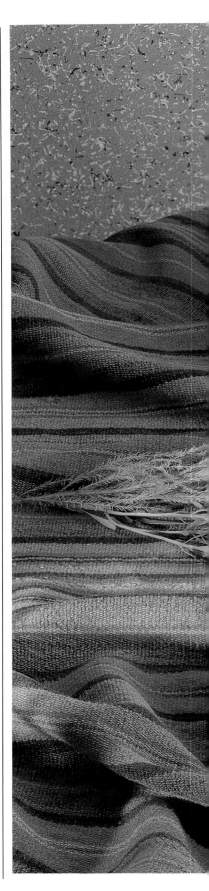

FROM THE TOP Sesame turkey with ginger and lychees; Soufflé cheese potatoes; Veal paupiettes

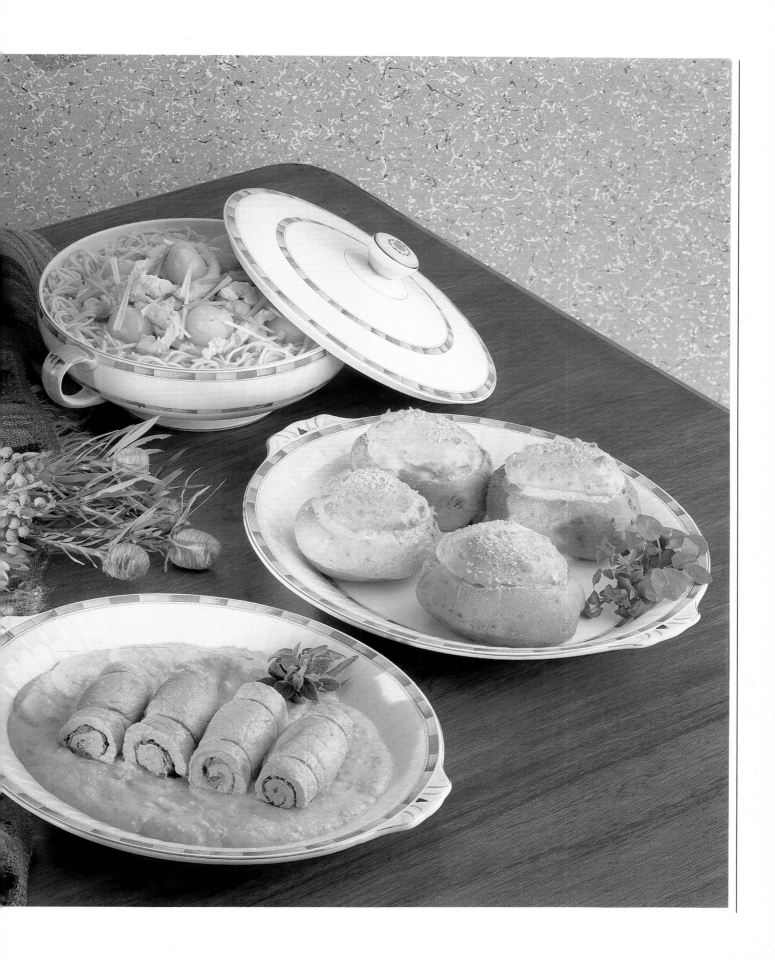

DECEMBER

Puddings

Mango Mousse

1 large ripe mango
1 tablespoon lime juice
300 ml (½ pint) unsweetened
* apple purée*
1 tablespoon clear honey
3 tablespoons plain
* unsweetened yogurt*
artificial sweetener, to taste
3 teaspoons powdered gelatine
2 tablespoons water
1 egg white

PREPARATION TIME:
30 minutes, plus chilling
CALORIES PER PORTION:
100 (420 kilojoules)

1. Halve the mango by cutting right round its circumference; remove the stone and scoop out the flesh into a bowl.
2. Blend the mango flesh and lime juice in the liquidizer; if necessary, make up to 300 ml (½ pint) with water.
3. Mix the mango and apple purées together; add the honey and yogurt. Add artificial sweetener to taste.
4. Put the gelatine and water into a small bowl; stand over a pan of hot water and stir until the gelatine has dissolved. Stir the gelatine mixture into the fruit purée.
5. Whisk the egg white until stiff but not dry; fold lightly but thoroughly into the mango and apple mixture.
6. Spoon into stemmed glasses and chill for 2–3 hours. (Can be chilled for up to 24 hours.)

Cranberry Sorbet

225 g (8 oz) fresh cranberries
300 ml (½ pint) unsweetened
* orange juice*
300 ml (½ pint) water
artificial sweetener, to taste
2 egg whites

PREPARATION TIME:
30 minutes, plus freezing
COOKING TIME:
30–40 minutes
CALORIES PER PORTION:
40 (170 kilojoules)

1. Put the cranberries into a pan with the orange juice and water; bring to the boil and simmer gently, covered, until the cranberries are tender.
2. Strain through a sieve, catching the cranberry juices in a bowl; blend the cooked cranberries in the liquidizer until smooth and add to the juices. Allow to cool and add sweetener to taste.
3. Pour the cranberry and orange mixture into a shallow container and freeze until 'slushy' around the edges. Whisk the egg whites until stiff but not dry.
4. Tip the semi-frozen sorbet into a bowl and break up the ice crystals; fold in the whisked egg whites. Return to the container and freeze until firm.
5. Scoop into pretty glasses and serve immediately.

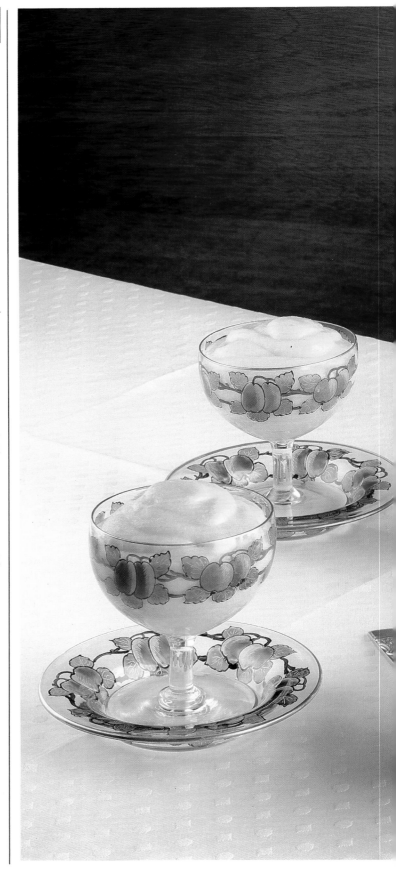

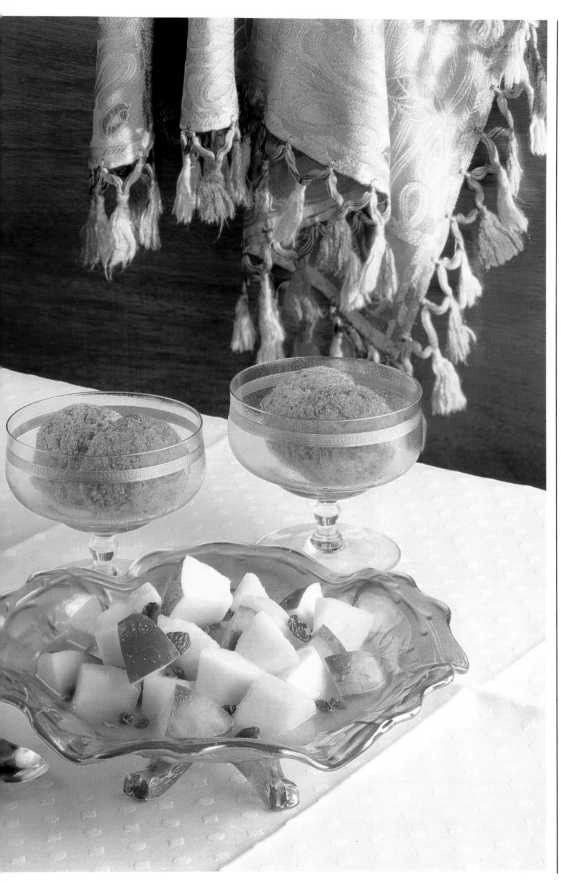

Orchard Salad

*4 ripe pears, peeled, halved
  and cored
300 ml (½ pint) apple juice
2 tablespoons lemon juice
2 red eating apples
1 tablespoon sultanas*

PREPARATION TIME:
30 minutes, plus chilling
CALORIES PER PORTION:
150 (630 kilojoules)

1. Put half the pears into a
liquidizer with the apple
juice; chop the remaining
pears and toss in the lemon
juice to prevent
discoloration.
2. Blend the pears and
apple juice together until
smooth and pour into a
glass bowl; add the
chopped pear and lemon
juice.
3. Halve, core and finely
chop the apples; combine
with the pear mixture and
add the sultanas.
4. Chill very well and serve
in small glass dessert
bowls.

FROM THE LEFT Mango mousse;
Cranberry sorbet; Orchard salad

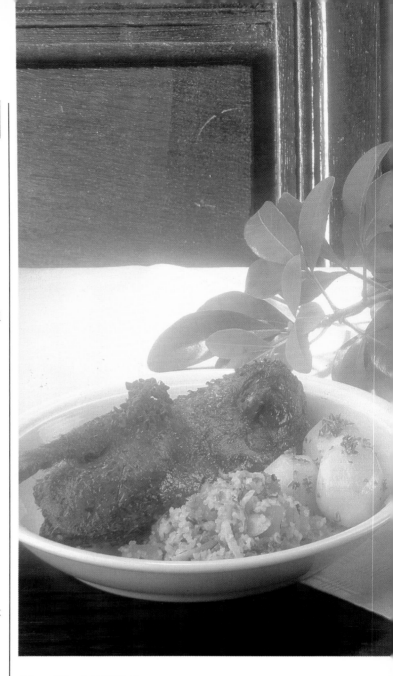

DECEMBER

Dinner Party for Six

Poached Scallops with Yogurt Sauce

6 scallops in their shells
Court bouillon:
300 ml (½ pint) white wine
300 ml (½ pint) water
1 onion, peeled and roughly chopped
1 celery stick, chopped
2 bay leaves
2–3 sprigs thyme
½ teaspoon salt
freshly ground black pepper
Yogurt sauce:
2 teaspoons mayonnaise
1 teaspoon mild French mustard
300 ml (½ pint) plain, unsweetened yogurt
6 needles of fresh rosemary, snipped and crushed with a little salt
3–4 drops lemon juice
To garnish:
½ crisp lettuce, shredded
6 anchovy fillets
3 black olives, stoned and sliced

PREPARATION TIME:
20 minutes, plus cooling
COOKING TIME:
about 10 minutes
CALORIES PER PORTION:
100 (420 kilojoules)

When buying scallops, ask the fishmonger to give you the deeper shell of the two they come in. Look for a brightly coloured roe (coral) and really firm white flesh.

1. Wash the scallops in cold water and if necessary cut off any black beard and intestine.
2. Combine the *court bouillon* ingredients and bring gently to the boil. Reduce to a simmer and poach the scallops in the liquid for 8 minutes. Strain the scallops and set aside to cool.
3. For the sauce, combine the mayonnaise and mustard. When blended, stir in the unsweetened yogurt. Stir in the crushed rosemary and finish with lemon juice and a grinding of pepper.
4. Assemble the dish just before serving. Make a nest of shredded lettuce in each shell and bed the scallops in the nests with the roe poking up. Spread the sauce over, leaving the roe and some of the lettuce exposed. Garnish with the anchovy fillets and black olive slices.

Stuffed Wild Duck

4 tablespoons boiling water
2 tablespoons bulgar (cracked wheat)
8 dried apricots, soaked overnight in cider and sliced
25 g (1 oz) flaked almonds, toasted
½ small cucumber, grated
1 tablespoon fresh thyme leaves
1 teaspoon salt
coarsely ground black pepper
3 wild ducks
sprigs of fresh thyme, to garnish

PREPARATION TIME:
20 minutes
COOKING TIME:
45–50 minutes
OVEN TEMPERATURE:
220°C, 425°F, Gas Mark 7
CALORIES PER PORTION:
430 (1800 kilojoules)

1. Pour the boiling water over the bulgar wheat to swell it.
2. When the wheat has absorbed the water, combine it with the other ingredients (except the ducks) and mix well.
3. Rub salt all over the ducks and spoon the

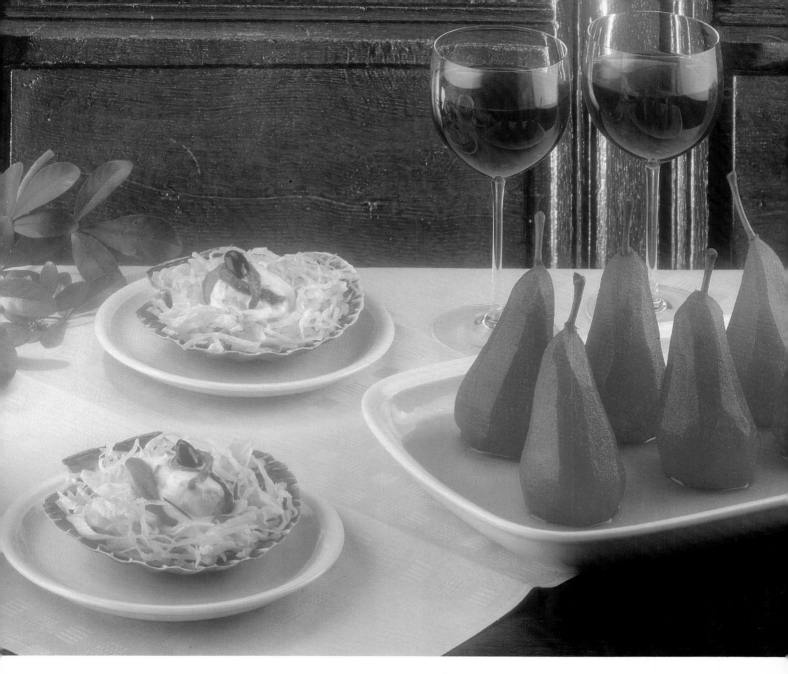

stuffing mixture into the cavity. Stand them on a wire rack in a large roasting tin, pour some water into the tin and roast in a preheated oven for 45–50 minutes.

4. To serve, halve the birds and garnish each half with a sprig of thyme. No sauce or gravy is needed as the stuffing is moist and so are the birds. Serve with steamed potatoes dressed with parsley and lemon juice and a simple green salad.

Pears in Claret

6 large Conference pears
600 ml (1 pint) claret
grated rind and juice of 1
  lemon
1 cinnamon stick
½ teaspoon nutmeg
25 g (1 oz) dark brown sugar

PREPARATION TIME:
20 minutes
COOKING TIME:
about 30–40 minutes
CALORIES PER PORTION:
105 (440 kilojoules)

1. Carefully peel the pears. Do not bother to remove the cores as they are small and quite tender. Cut a slice off the bottom of each pear so it will stand up.

2. Put the claret in a saucepan just big enough for the pears to fit in side by side, standing up.

3. Add the lemon rind and juice to the claret along with the cinnamon, nutmeg and sugar. Bring to simmering point and add the pears (if the pears are not completely immersed add cold water as necessary). Cover and simmer for about 30–40 minutes or until the pears are softened.

4. Carefully lift the pears out of the pan into a serving dish or individual dishes. Boil the liquid left in the pan fast to reduce by half, then spoon some of the thickened liquid over the pears to glaze. Serve either hot or cold.

FROM THE LEFT Stuffed wild duck; Poached scallops with yogurt sauce; Pears in claret

JANUARY

New Year's Eve Dinner for Ten

With this meal, you could serve a little very dry white wine with the terrine (mix it with sparkling mineral water if you like), nothing with the sorbet and a light claret with the partridges. A rosé champagne to accompany the dessert and to greet the New Year would be wonderful.

Fish Terrine

225 g (8 oz) smoked salmon
  offcuts
1 teaspoon Dijon mustard
2 tablespoons lemon juice
½ teaspoon sugar
½ teaspoon dried dill
3 egg whites
150 ml (¼ pint) single cream
450 g (1 lb) skinned and
  boned bream or haddock, cut
  into chunks
2 tablespoons chopped fresh
  parsley
salt
white pepper
1 egg yolk
150 ml (¼ pint) plain
  unsweetened yogurt
1 red pepper, blanched,
  seeded and finely shredded
5 slices wholemeal toast, cut
  into triangles, to serve

PREPARATION TIME:
1 hour, plus chilling
COOKING TIME:
1–1½ hours
OVEN TEMPERATURE:
140°C, 275°F, Gas Mark 1
CALORIES PER PORTION:
130 (545 kilojoules)

1. Purée the smoked salmon adding the mustard, lemon juice, sugar, dill and 1 egg white.
2. Stand a bowl over ice and turn the salmon into it. Mix in the cream, a dribble at a time. When it is all incorporated, cover the bowl and chill while you prepare the bream.
3. Purée the bream in a food processor adding the parsley, salt and white pepper to taste, and the remaining egg whites.
4. Place the mixture in a bowl over ice. Mix the egg yolk with the yogurt and combine with the puréed bream.
5. Line a 1 kg (2 lb) loaf tin or equivalent size terrine with non-stick silicone paper. Spread the bream mixture in the bottom, cover with the shredded red pepper and then the salmon mixture. Smooth the surface and cover with 2 layers of non-stick silicone paper.
6. Place in a roasting tin half-filled with water in a preheated oven for 1–1½ hours (a skewer should come out clean when it is cooked). Allow to cool, then chill for 12 hours.
7. Turn out, peel off the paper and serve in slices with toast.

Lemon and Orange Sorbet

225 g (8 oz) sugar
600 ml (1 pint) water
150 ml (¼ pint) lemon juice
750 ml (1¼ pints)
  unsweetened orange juice
1 teaspoon Angostura bitters
4 egg whites

PREPARATION TIME:
15 minutes, plus freezing
COOKING TIME:
10 minutes
CALORIES PER
DESSERTSPOON:
60 (250 kilojoules)

A very small portion of this sorbet should be served between courses to cleanse the palate; no more than a rounded dessertspoon per person. Return the remaining sorbet to the freezer to serve at a later date.

1. Set the refrigerator or freezer to its coldest setting and chill all the utensils you need to make the sorbet.
2. Make a syrup by boiling the sugar in the water with 1 tablespoon of the lemon juice for 10 minutes.
3. Strain the fruit juices, mix with the sugar syrup and add the Angostura bitters.

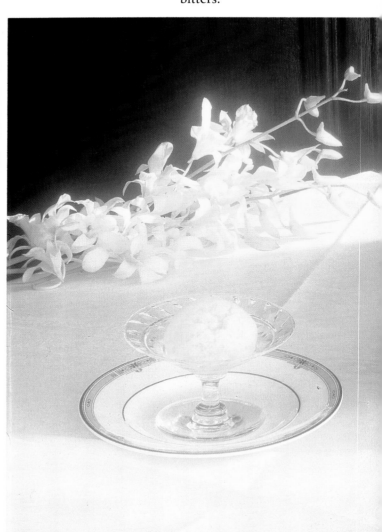

4. Freeze as fast as possible, whisking thoroughly at intervals until the mixture is quite firm. Continue to freeze without any further stirring.

5. Whip the egg whites until stiff but not dry.

6. Remove the sorbet from the freezer and tip into a well chilled bowl. Break down the ice with a fork and fold in the egg whites.

7. Return to the freezer until solid. Serve one rounded dessertspoonful per person.

FROM THE LEFT Lemon and orange sorbet; Fish terrine; Partridge with pears

Partridge with Pears

1 sprig fresh rosemary
2 bay leaves
10 cloves
300 ml (½ pint) dry white wine
300 ml (½ pint) water
10 partridges
salt
1 lemon, quartered
10 firm pears, peeled

PREPARATION TIME:
30 minutes
COOKING TIME:
55–60 minutes or 1 hour 25 minutes
OVEN TEMPERATURE:
200°C, 400°F, Gas Mark 6
CALORIES PER PORTION:
850 (1465 kilojoules)

1. Put the herbs and cloves in a saucepan with the wine and water, bring to the boil, cover and remove from the heat while you prepare the birds.

2. Rub each bird inside and out with salt and a cut lemon. Arrange them in two earthenware oven-to-table dishes, then arrange the pears around the birds.

3. Bring the wine and water to the boil again quickly and pour over the birds and pears. Place in a preheated oven. Cook for 45–50 minutes if both dishes fit on the centre shelf. If not, put the dishes on different shelves for 20 minutes, then swap them for the next 20 minutes.

Change them over again for a further 15 minutes, then take the top dish out and keep it warm while you give the other dish a final 20 minutes in the centre of the oven. During cooking, check that the liquids do not dry up, topping up with more water if the need arises.

4. Serve one pear and a little of the cooking juice with each partridge. Accompany with red cabbage flavoured with juniper berries and steamed potatoes.

Menu continues over page

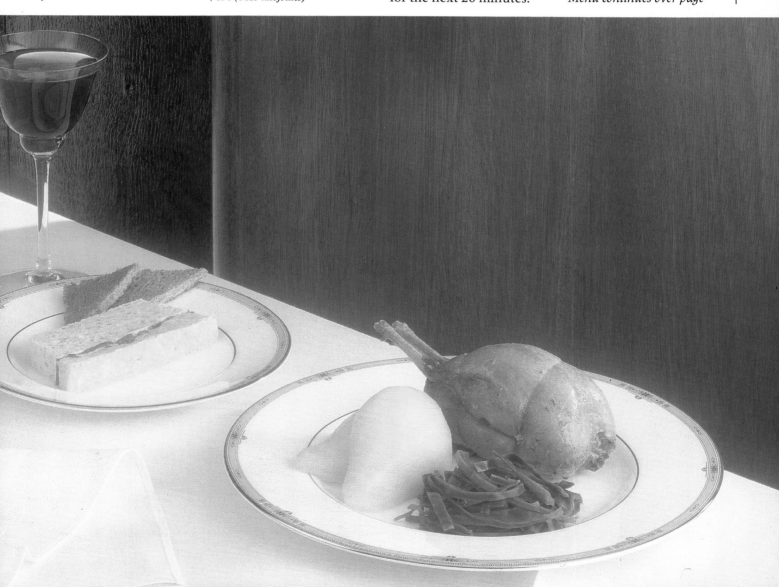

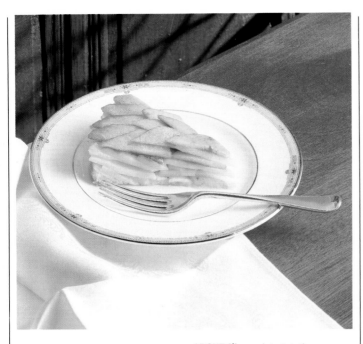

ABOVE Slimmer's tarte tatin

JANUARY

Hors d'oeuvres and Light Meals

Slimmer's Tarte Tatin

1.25 kg (2¾ lb) green eating
  apples
1 teaspoon ground cinnamon
15 g (½oz) molasses sugar
1 egg, separated
15 g (½ oz) sugar
2 drops vanilla essence
20 g (¾ oz) plain flour, sieved

PREPARATION TIME:
about 1 hour
COOKING TIME:
30–40 minutes
OVEN TEMPERATURE:
200°C, 400°F, Gas Mark 6
CALORIES PER PORTION:
110 (440 kilojoules)

1. Have ready a basin of
salted water to put the
peeled apples in to prevent
discoloration. Peel, core
and quarter the apples,
then slice them as finely as
possible.
2. Mix the cinnamon with
the molasses sugar.
3. Line the base of a 20 cm
(8 inch) loose-bottomed
cake tin with non-stick
silicone paper and spread
half the sugar and
cinnamon over.

4. Carefully arrange the
apple slices, slightly overlapping, in an ever
decreasing circle on the
bottom of the tin. The layer
of sugar should be
completely covered.
5. Repeat the process until
you have used up a little
more than half the apples,
then spread the remaining
sugar and cinnamon over.
Continue with the apples
until all are used. Press
down lightly.
6. Cream the egg yolk with
the sugar until light and
creamy. Add the vanilla.
7. Whip the egg white until
stiff and fold it in, then
carefully fold in the flour.
Spread this mixture on top
of the apples, pressing
them down if necessary.
8. Place in a preheated
oven for 20 minutes, then
check that the sponge
topping is not colouring
too fast; if necessary cover
with a piece of silicone
paper. Continue cooking
for another 15 minutes.
9. Just before serving,
carefully invert on to a
plate. Peel off the paper
and serve warm or cold.

Smoked Cod Kedgeree

225 g (8 oz) brown rice
salt
1 small onion, peeled and
  finely chopped
20 g (¾ oz) butter
2 tablespoons plain
  unsweetened yogurt
175 g (6 oz) smoked cod,
  flaked
1 hard-boiled egg, roughly
  chopped
2 tablespoons chopped fresh
  parsley
freshly ground black pepper
paprika, to garnish

PREPARATION TIME:
20 minutes
COOKING TIME:
about 35 minutes
CALORIES PER PORTION:
365 (1530 kilojoules)

1. Cook the brown rice in
boiling salted water for
about 25 minutes until just
tender. Drain thoroughly.
2. Fry the onion gently in
the butter for 3–4 minutes.
Add the drained cooked
rice, and stir over the heat
for a further 2–3 minutes,
until the rice is coated.
3. Add the yogurt, fish,
chopped egg, chopped
parsley and pepper to
taste; stir over the heat for
1–2 minutes, until all the
ingredients are heated
through.
4. Serve, garnished with
paprika.

Minced Chicken Mimosa

2 boned chicken breasts,
  about 150 g (5 oz) each
150 ml (¼ pint) chicken stock
150 ml (¼ pint) dry white
  wine
salt
freshly ground black pepper
1 tablespoon chopped fresh
  chives
2 tablespoons olive oil
2 tablespoons tarragon
  vinegar
1 garlic clove, peeled and
  crushed
To serve:
1 hard-boiled egg
2 slices wholemeal toast, cut
  into fingers or triangles

PREPARATION TIME:
25 minutes, plus chilling
COOKING TIME:
15–20 minutes
CALORIES PER PORTION:
255 (1065 kilojoules)

1. Put the chicken breasts
into a shallow pan with the
stock, white wine and salt
and pepper to taste. Cover
and simmer gently for
about 15 minutes until the
chicken is just tender.
Remove the chicken
breasts with a slotted
spoon and allow to cool
slightly.
2. Chop the chicken
roughly and put through
the fine blade of the
mincer; mix with the
chopped chives.

3. Mix the olive oil with the tarragon vinegar, garlic, and salt and pepper to taste; stir into the minced chicken and chives. Chill for 1 hour.
4. Separate the white and yolk of the hard-boiled egg; chop the white finely and sieve the yolk.
5. Spoon the minced chicken on to small serving plates, and garnish with the egg white and yolk.
6. Serve with wholemeal toast.

Spiced Carrot Soup

1 medium onion, peeled and finely chopped
1 tablespoon olive oil
450 g (1 lb) carrots, peeled and roughly chopped
1 slice fresh ginger, 5 mm (¼ inch) thick
generous pinch of mixed spice
1 teaspoon grated orange rind
600 ml (1 pint) chicken stock
300 ml (½ pint) skimmed milk
1 teaspoon chopped fresh coriander
To garnish:
carrot slivers
fresh coriander leaves

PREPARATION TIME:
20 minutes
COOKING TIME:
about 30 minutes
CALORIES PER PORTION:
95 (400 kilojoules)

1. Fry the onion gently in the oil for 3 minutes; add the carrots and fry together for a further 2−3 minutes.
2. Squeeze the fresh ginger in a garlic press and add the juice to the vegetables; add the mixed spice, orange rind, stock, skimmed milk and chopped coriander.
3. Cover, bring to the boil and simmer gently for about 20 minutes, until the carrots are tender.
4. Blend the soup in a liquidizer until smooth.
5. Reheat the soup, adjusting the texture with a little extra stock if desired, then ladle into soup bowls and garnish with carrot slivers and sprigs of coriander.

CLOCKWISE FROM LEFT Spiced carrot soup; Smoked cod kedgeree; Minced chicken mimosa

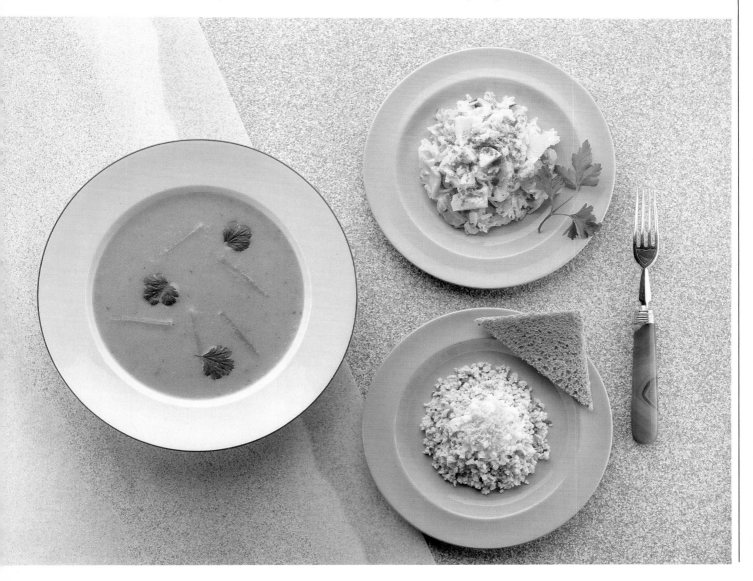

JANUARY

Main Courses

Stir-Fried Crab and Sole

25 g (1 oz) butter
2 tablespoons olive oil
1 small onion, peeled and
   finely chopped
1 garlic clove, peeled and
   crushed
2 leeks, cleaned and cut into
   julienne strips
350 g (12 oz) sole fillets,
   skinned and cut into thin
   strips
225 (8 oz) white crabmeat,
   flaked
4 tablespoons chicken stock
1 small avocado pear, peeled,
   halved, stoned and sliced
1 teaspoon grated lemon rind
salt
1 teaspoon green peppercorns
   in brine
2 tablespoons finely chopped
   fresh parsley or dill, to
   garnish

PREPARATION TIME:
15 minutes
COOKING TIME:
10–13 minutes
CALORIES PER PORTION:
260 (1090 kilojoules)

1. Heat the butter and oil
in a wok or large frying
pan and gently fry the
onion and garlic for 3
minutes.
2. Add the julienne strips
of leek and the strips of
sole, and stir-fry gently
until the fish is opaque.
3. Add the crabmeat, stock,
avocado slices, lemon rind,
salt and peppercorns; stir-
fry for 2–3 minutes.
4. Serve immediately,
sprinkled with parsley.

Veal with Olives

2 tablespoons olive oil
4 veal noisettes, trimmed of
   fat, about 150 g (5 oz) each
1 small onion, peeled and
   thinly sliced
1 bay leaf
1 strip lemon peel
300 ml (½ pint) white wine
50 g (2 oz) green olives, pitted
1 teaspoon fresh thyme
salt
freshly ground black pepper
3 tablespoons plain
   unsweetened yogurt
1 egg yolk
To garnish:
8 large green olives
sprigs of fresh thyme

PREPARATION TIME:
10 minutes
COOKING TIME:
30–35 minutes
CALORIES PER PORTION:
315 (1320 kilojoules)

1. Heat the olive oil and
gently fry the noisettes
until lightly golden.
2. Add the onion, bay leaf,
lemon peel, white wine,
pitted green olives and
thyme with salt and
pepper to taste.
3. Cover and simmer for 25
minutes, until tender.
Remove and keep warm.
4. Blend the cooking
liquid, minus the bay leaf,
with the yogurt and egg
yolk. Heat the sauce
through very gently
without boiling.
5. Spoon the hot sauce
over the veal and garnish
with the olives and sprigs
of thyme. Serve with new
potatoes and carrots.

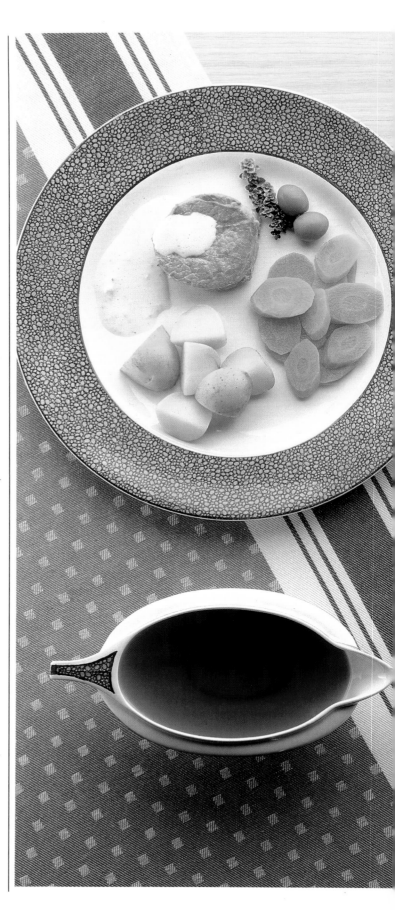

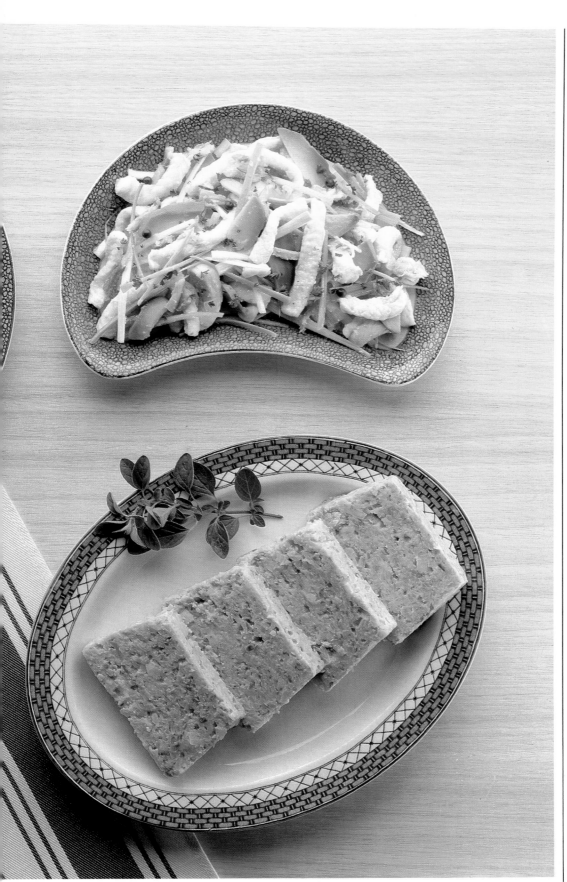

Cheese and Lentil Loaf

175 g (6 oz) lentils, soaked
  overnight
1 garlic clove, peeled and
  crushed
1 small onion, peeled and
  finely chopped
1 green pepper, cored and
  chopped
50 g (2 oz) well-flavoured
  cheese, grated
2 tablespoons grated
  Parmesan cheese
2 tablespoons chopped fresh
  parsley
2 eggs, beaten
beef consommé
1 teaspoon French mustard
salt
freshly ground black pepper

PREPARATION TIME:
25 minutes
COOKING TIME:
about 1½ hours
OVEN TEMPERATURE:
180°C, 350°F, Gas Mark 4
CALORIES PER SLICE
(MAKES 8 SLICES):
260 (670 kilojoules)

1. Drain the lentils and put
in a pan with water to
cover; add the garlic. Bring
to the boil and simmer for
20–30 minutes, until
tender. Drain thoroughly.
2. Mix the cooked lentils
with the chopped onion,
green pepper, cheeses,
parsley, beaten eggs, 3
tablespoons consommé,
mustard, and salt and
pepper to taste.
3. Put the mixture into a
greased and lined 450 g
(1 lb) loaf tin. Cover with
lightly greased foil. Bake in
a preheated oven for 1 hour.
4. Allow the loaf to cool for
a few minutes in its tin.
5. Turn out and serve with
more warmed beef
consommé.

CLOCKWISE FROM LEFT Veal with
olives; Stir-fried crab and sole; Cheese
and lentil loaf

JANUARY

Puddings

Two Fruits Compote

300 ml (½ pint) unsweetened orange juice
4 tablespoons lemon juice
2 tablespoons low calorie apricot jam
3 firm pears, peeled, halved, cored and cut into sections
8 apricots, blanched and skinned
twists of orange peel, to decorate (optional)

PREPARATION TIME:
10–15 minutes
COOKING TIME:
about 20 minutes
CALORIES PER PORTION:
130 (545 kilojoules)

1. Put the orange juice, lemon juice and apricot jam into a pan; stir over a gentle heat until the jam has dissolved.
2. Add the prepared fruits to the syrup; cover the pan, bring to the boil and simmer gently for about 12–15 minutes, until the pears are tender. Cool slightly.
3. Spoon into one large or 4 small dishes (heatproof ones if the compote is very hot), and decorate with a twist of orange peel if liked.

Grape and White Wine Jelly

4 teaspoons powdered gelatine
300 ml (½ pint) apple juice
300 ml (½ pint) dry white wine
225 g (8 oz) green grapes, skinned, halved and seeded
clusters of green grapes, to decorate

PREPARATION TIME:
about 25 minutes, plus chilling
CALORIES PER PORTION:
135 (560 kilojoules)

1. Place the gelatine and 3 tablespoons of the apple juice in a small bowl. Stand in a saucepan of hot water and stir over a gentle heat until dissolved. Combine with the remaining apple juice and white wine and put to one side until syrupy.
2. Lightly oil one 900 ml (1½ pint) mould, or 4 small ones.
3. Stir the prepared grapes into the syrupy jelly and pour into the mould.
4. Chill for about 2–3 hours, until set.
5. Carefully turn out the jelly on to a serving plate and decorate with small clusters of grapes.

Apple Lime Crunch

450 g (1 lb) cooking apples, peeled, cored and sliced
2 tablespoons freshly squeezed lime juice
2 tablespoons water
artificial sweetener, to taste
1 egg, separated
4 tablespoons muesli, lightly toasted
4 teaspoons lime curd or lime marmalade
4 thin slices of lime, to decorate

PREPARATION TIME:
20–25 minutes, plus chilling
COOKING TIME:
about 5 minutes
CALORIES PER PORTION:
150 (620 kilojoules)

1. Put the apples into a pan with the lime juice and water; cover and simmer gently until the apples are soft and pulpy. Add artificial sweetener to taste. Chill.
2. Beat the egg yolk into the cooked apple; whisk the egg white until stiff but not dry, and fold lightly but thoroughly into the apple mixture.
3. Put half the apple mixture into 4 tall glasses, and sprinkle the toasted muesli over the top. Add a spoonful of lime curd or lime marmalade and top up with the remaining apple mixture.
4. Decorate each one with a twisted lime slice, and serve immediately.

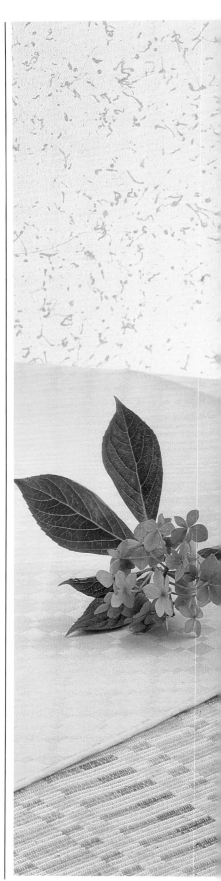

FROM THE RIGHT Apple lime crunch; Grape and white wine jelly; Two fruits compote

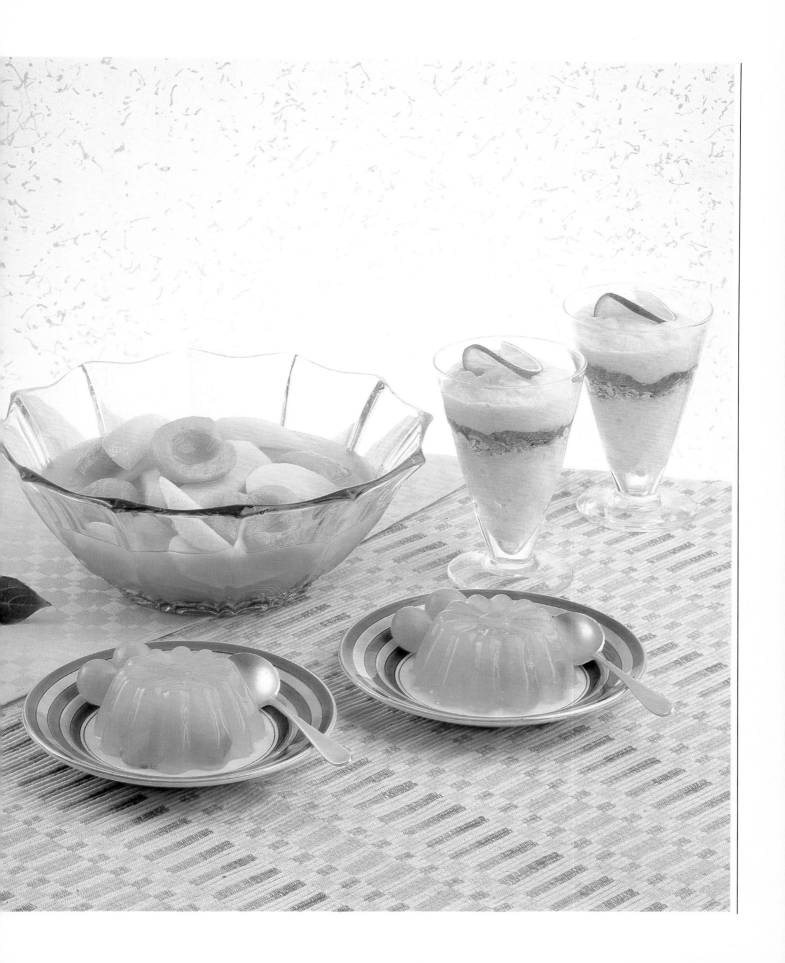

JANUARY

Dinner Party for Six

Fennel à la Grecque

2 tablespoons olive oil
1 teaspoon coriander seed
1 bay leaf
4 sprigs fresh parsley
1 celery stick, finely chopped
3 cloves
½ teaspoon green peppercorns
  in brine
4 small fennel bulbs, trimmed
  and quartered
2 tablespoons lemon juice
200 ml (7 fl oz) white wine
200 ml (7 fl oz) water
½ teaspoon sugar
salt

PREPARATION TIME:
10 minutes
COOKING TIME:
about 45 minutes
CALORIES PER PORTION:
75 (315 kilojoules)

1. Heat the oil, add the
coriander and fry for a few
seconds before adding the
bay leaf, parsley, celery,
cloves and peppercorns.
2. Cook for 1 minute, then
add the fennel, lemon
juice, wine and water.
Bring to the boil, add the
sugar and salt, cover and
simmer for 40 minutes.
3. Transfer the fennel to a
serving dish. Bring the
liquids in the pan to the
boil and reduce by half,
then strain over the fennel,
cool and chill. Serve at
room temperature.

Beef and Artichokes

1 kg (2 lb) lean chuck steak,
  cut into cubes
½ teaspoon allspice
½ teaspoon ground cinnamon
½ teaspoon salt
coarsely ground black pepper
4 garlic cloves, peeled
8 tablespoons red wine
1 tablespoon oil
½ teaspoon ground cumin
750 g (1½ lb) Jerusalem
  artichokes, blanched and
  scraped, cut into chunks

PREPARATION TIME:
15 minutes, plus marinating
COOKING TIME:
1 hour 10 minutes
CALORIES PER PORTION:
265 (1110 kilojoules)

1. Put the meat in a bowl
and sprinkle over the
allspice, cinnamon, salt
and pepper. Add 2 of the
garlic cloves, chopped.
2. Pour over the wine and
mix well. Cover and leave
to marinate for at least 4
hours (not more than 24).
3. Heat the oil and fry the
remaining garlic, halved,
with the cumin.
4. Strain the meat and add
to pan, reserving marinade.
5. Seal the meat over a
high heat, then transfer to
a flameproof casserole.
6. Add the artichokes and
marinade, cover and
simmer for 1 hour.

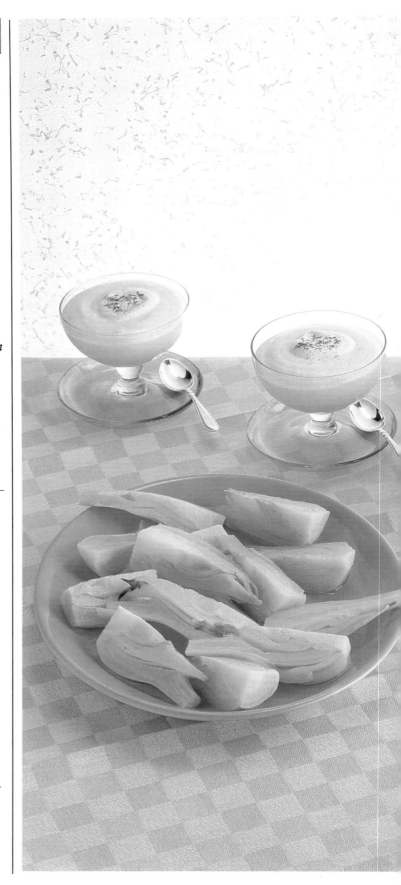

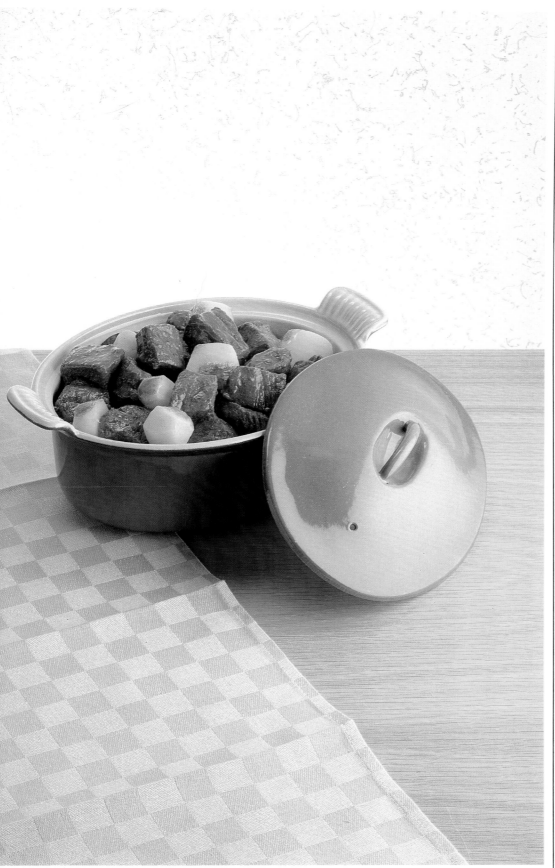

Greek Syllabub

65 ml (2½ fl oz) whipping
  cream
3 tablespoons lemon juice
3 teaspoons light tahini
  (sesame seed paste)
1 tablespoon clear honey
  (preferably Hymetus)
600 ml (1 pint) plain
  unsweetened yogurt
2 egg whites
ground cinnamon, for
  sprinkling

PREPARATION TIME:
15 minutes
CALORIES PER PORTION:
120 (500 kilojoules)

1. Whip the cream until it
no longer runs when the
bowl is tipped; it should
move very slowly.
2. In another bowl stir the
lemon juice into the tahini
paste and whisk it with a
fork until it is well blended.
Stir in the honey.
3. Combine this mixture
with the whipped cream,
then add the yogurt.
4. Whisk the egg whites
stiffly and fold in.
5. Divide the syllabub
between 6 tall glasses and
sprinkle each with a little
cinnamon before serving.

CLOCKWISE FROM RIGHT Beef and
artichokes; Fennel à la grecque; Greek
syllabub

FEBRUARY

St.Valentine's Dinner for Two

A luxurious menu that requires the minimum of last minute cooking, so that you can relax and enjoy the company of your Valentine.

Dutch Avocado

1 small avocado pear
2 tablespoons lemon juice
1 eating apple
25 g (1 oz) sultanas
1 teaspoon mild curry powder
2 tablespoons plain
* unsweetened yogurt*
salt
freshly ground black pepper

PREPARATION TIME:
15–20 minutes
CALORIES PER PORTION:
240 (1010 kilojoules)

1. Halve and stone the avocado; score the flesh into small squares, cutting through almost to the skin, and scoop it out into a bowl; sprinkle with ½ tablespoon lemon juice.
2. Peel and core the apple and cut into cubes the same size as the avocado. Soak the sultanas in the remaining lemon juice for 5 minutes. Combine the avocado, apple and sultanas.
3. Mix the curry powder with the yogurt and combine with the apple and avocado, add salt and pepper and pile into the avocado skins.
4. Serve immediately or cover tightly with cling film and chill until ready to serve.

Spinach-Stuffed Lamb

225 g (8 oz) fresh or frozen
* spinach, cooked, drained*
* very well and chopped*
15 g (½ oz) fresh mint, finely
* chopped*
4 garlic cloves, peeled and
* finely chopped*
1 teaspoon vinegar
pinch of sugar
salt
freshly ground black pepper
½ small boned leg of lamb
* (knuckle end), about 400 g*
* (14 oz) (see below)*
175 ml (6 fl oz) red wine
sprigs of fresh mint, to
* garnish*

PREPARATION TIME:
20 minutes
COOKING TIME:
45–60 minutes
OVEN TEMPERATURE:
180°C, 350°F, Gas Mark 4
CALORIES PER PORTION:
210 (880 kilojoules)

At this time of year imported lamb is at its best and least fatty. Ask the butcher to remove the bone but do not let him roll it. You should end up with a roughly triangular piece of meat. The cooking time will depend upon whether you like your lamb well done or pink.

1. Mix the spinach with the mint, garlic, vinegar, sugar and add salt and pepper to taste.
2. Trim every scrap of fat off the lamb. Lay it out flat with the boned side up and spread the spinach mixture over. Fold the meat over and secure with string as if tying a parcel.
3. Lay the meat in a roasting dish or pan and pour over the red wine, adding a little water if the pan is much larger than the meat. Cook in a preheated oven for 45–55 minutes.
4. Transfer to a hot carving platter and cut into thick slices. Pour off excess fat from the roasting pan and pour the remaining juices over the lamb slices.
5. Serve immediately with rice, garnishing the slices with fresh mint.

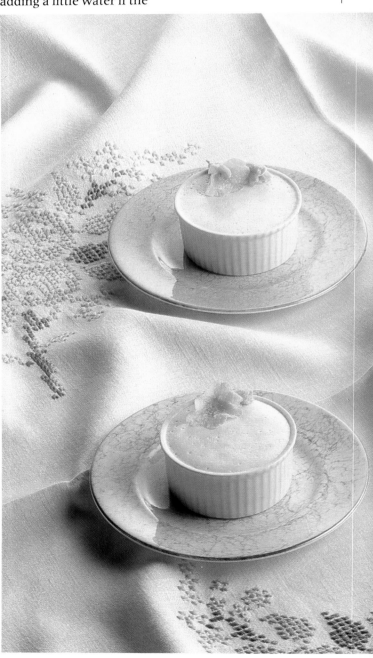

Little Lemon Mousse Soufflés

1 sachet powdered gelatine
4 tablespoons lemon juice
grated rind of 1 lemon
25 g (1 oz) caster sugar
1 egg, separated
3 tablespoons plain
  unsweetened yogurt
1 egg white (size 1)
frosted primroses, to decorate
  (page 89)

PREPARATION TIME:
20 minutes
COOKING TIME:
3–5 minutes
CALORIES PER PORTION:
120 (500 kilojoules)

1. Place the gelatine and lemon juice in a small bowl. Stand in a pan of hot water and stir over a very gentle heat until dissolved.
2. Pound the lemon rind with the sugar, then cream it with the egg yolk. When it is light and frothy, slowly whisk in the dissolved gelatine. Cool completely, then stir in the yogurt.
3. Whisk the egg whites until stiff and carefully fold them in. Spoon into tall glasses or small ramekins and chill until set.
4. Decorate each soufflé with a frosted primrose just before serving.

CLOCKWISE FROM TOP Spinach-stuffed lamb; Dutch avocado; Little lemon mousse soufflés

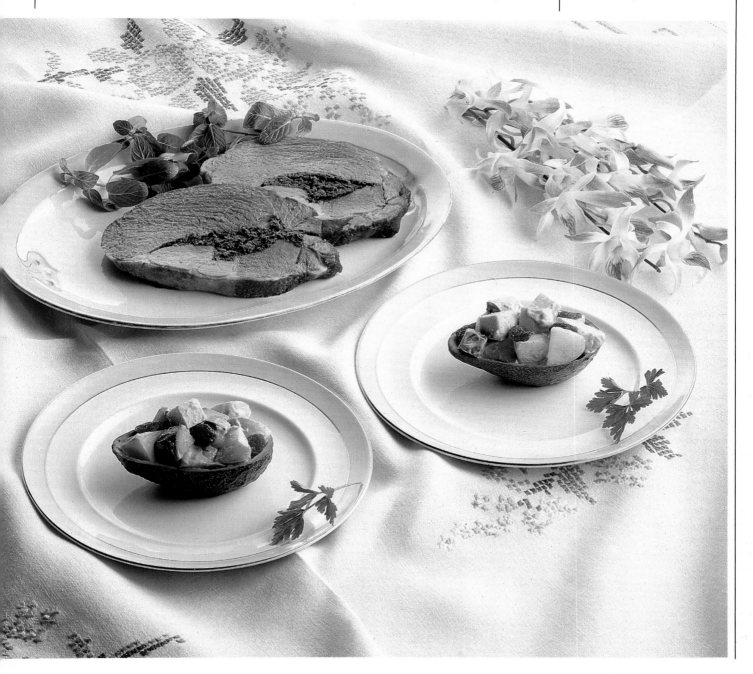

FEBRUARY

Hors d'oeuvres and Light Meals

Egg and Mushroom Cocottes

15 g (½ oz) butter
100 g (4 oz) button
  mushrooms, sliced
2 teaspoons lemon juice
2 teaspoons Worcestershire
  sauce
salt
freshly ground black pepper
1 tablespoon finely chopped
  fresh parsley
4 eggs
To serve:
2 teaspoons chopped fresh
  thyme
2 slices wholemeal bread,
  thinly spread with low fat
  spread and cut into fingers

PREPARATION TIME:
about 15 minutes
COOKING TIME:
15–20 minutes
OVEN TEMPERATURE:
180°C, 350°F, Gas Mark 4
CALORIES PER PORTION:
150 (620 kilojoules)

1. Heat the butter and the mushrooms gently with the lemon juice and Worcestershire sauce for 3–4 minutes.
2. Add salt and pepper to taste and the parsley; spoon into 4 lightly greased cocotte dishes.
3. Carefully crack an egg into each dish then cover each one with a small circle of foil, pinching the edges to seal.
4. Stand the cocottes in a roasting tin and add hot water to come half-way up the sides.
5. Bake in a preheated oven for 12–15 minutes, until the eggs are just set.
6. Sprinkle with thyme and serve with the bread.

Aubergine and Lumpfish Purée

1 large aubergine
3 tablespoons plain
  unsweetened yogurt
2 tablespoons chopped fresh
  parsley
1 tablespoon chopped fresh
  chives
2 garlic cloves, peeled and
  crushed
4 tablespoons lemon juice
salt
freshly ground black pepper
2 tablespoons sesame seeds
To serve:
2 tablespoons black or orange
  lumpfish roe
4 slices black pumpernickel,
  cut into squares
chopped fresh chives, to
  garnish

PREPARATION TIME:
15–20 minutes, plus chilling
COOKING TIME:
8–10 minutes
OVEN TEMPERATURE:
200°C, 400°F, Gas Mark 6
CALORIES PER PORTION:
190 (760 kilojoules)

1. Char the aubergine either by baking it whole in the oven, or putting it under a preheated grill. (If it is grilled it will need turning regularly.) The aubergine skin should be blistered and wrinkled and the flesh inside should be soft. Allow to cool.
2. Scoop out all the aubergine flesh and squeeze gently in a piece of clean muslin to get rid of

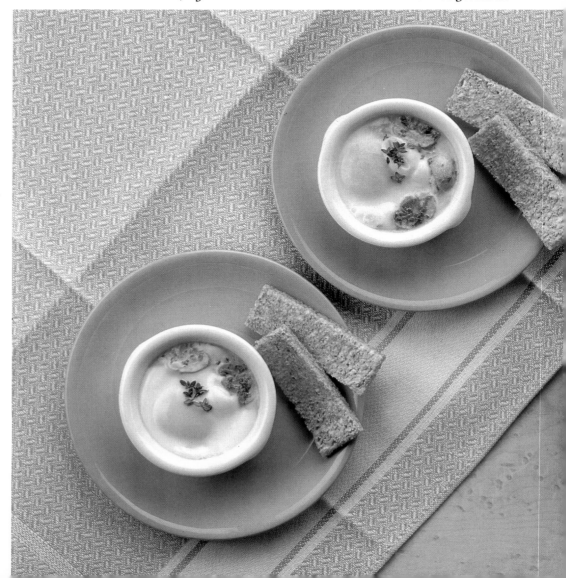

any bitter juices. (Do not squeeze tightly.)

3. Blend the aubergine flesh to a purée in a liquidizer or food processor; add the yogurt, parsley, chives, garlic, lemon juice and salt and pepper to taste. Blend once again until smooth.

4. Stir the sesame seeds into the purée; cover and chill for 1–2 hours.

5. Spoon the purée on to small plates; make a 'well' in each portion and fill with lumpfish roe.

6. Sprinkle each portion with chopped chives and serve with the pumpernickel squares.

Fish and Leek Soup

1 small onion, thinly sliced
1 garlic clove, peeled and
  crushed
2 tablespoons olive oil
2 medium leeks, cleaned and
  cut into fine strips
2 tablespoons chopped fresh
  parsley
225 g (8 oz) white fish fillet,
  cubed
300 ml (½ pint) chicken stock
300 ml (½ pint) skimmed
  milk
salt
freshly ground black pepper
3 tablespoons plain
  unsweetened yogurt
1 egg yolk
1 tablespoon finely chopped
  green pepper, to garnish

PREPARATION TIME:
10 minutes
COOKING TIME:
about 20 minutes
CALORIES PER PORTION
190 (790 kilojoules)

1. Fry the onion and garlic gently in the olive oil for 3 minutes; add the leeks and parsley and fry for a further 3 minutes.

2. Add the cubed fish, stock, skimmed milk and salt and pepper to taste; bring to the boil and simmer gently for 10 minutes.

3. Beat the yogurt and egg yolk together. Blend with a little of the hot soup and then add to the remaining soup in the pan.

4. Heat through gently, without boiling, for 1–2 minutes.

5. Serve piping hot, garnished with finely chopped green pepper.

FROM THE LEFT Egg and mushroom cocottes; Fish and leek soup; Aubergine and lumpfish purée

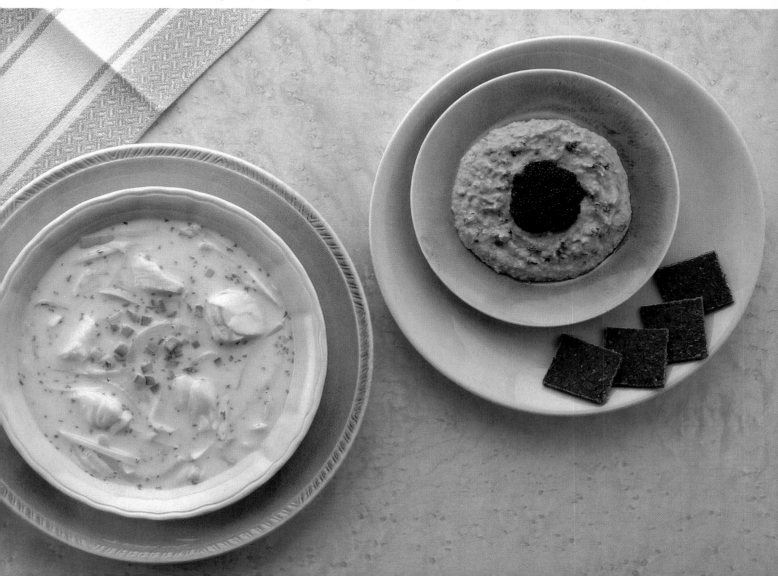

FEBRUARY

Main Courses

Smoked Haddock and Celery Risotto

1 tablespoon olive oil
1 medium onion, peeled and
  finely chopped
1 garlic clove, peeled and
  crushed
225 g (8 oz) long-grain rice
750 ml (1¼ pints) chicken
  stock
salt
freshly ground black pepper
350 g (12 oz) smoked haddock
  fillet, cut into thin strips
2 celery sticks, finely shredded
To garnish:
1 hard-boiled egg yolk
1 tablespoon chopped fresh
  chives

PREPARATION TIME:
15 minutes
COOKING TIME:
about 30 minutes
CALORIES PER PORTION:
360 (1510 kilojoules)

1. Heat the oil and fry the
onion gently for 3
minutes; add the garlic and
rice and fry gently until the
rice is opaque and evenly
coated with oil.
2. Gradually stir in the
stock and add salt and
pepper to taste; cover and
simmer for 10 minutes.
3. Add the strips of smoked
haddock and the celery;
cover and simmer gently for
a further 10–15 minutes,
until the fish, vegetables
and rice are all tender.
4. Sieve the egg yolk.
5. Spoon the risotto into a
dish and garnish with the
egg yolk and chives.

Chilli Beef

1 tablespoon olive oil
1 small onion, peeled and
  finely chopped
1 garlic clove, peeled and
  crushed
450 g (1 lb) lean minced beef
1 tablespoon chilli powder (or
  to taste)
1 tablespoon tomato purée
300 ml (½ pint) beef stock
6 tomatoes, skinned, seeded
  and chopped
1 small red pepper, cored and
  chopped
1 × 225 g (8 oz) can kidney
  beans, rinsed and drained
To garnish:
4 tablespoons plain
  unsweetened yogurt
chilli powder (optional)

PREPARATION TIME:
10–15 minutes
COOKING TIME:
about 30 minutes
CALORIES PER PORTION:
375 (1560 kilojoules)

1. Heat the oil and fry the
onion gently for 3
minutes; add the garlic and
beef and fry until browned.
2. Stir in the chilli powder
and cook for 1 minute.
3. Add the tomato purée,
beef stock, tomatoes,
chopped red pepper and
kidney beans; cover and
simmer gently for 20–25
minutes, until the minced
beef is tender.
4. Spoon the mince on to
hot plates and place a
tablespoon of yogurt next
to it. Sprinkle a little chilli
powder over the yogurt.
5. Serve immediately with
rice or a salad.

Pancakes with Celery and Peanuts

50 g (2 oz) wholemeal flour
pinch of salt
1 egg
150 ml (¼ pint) skimmed
  milk and water mixed
1 tablespoon chopped fresh
  parsley
olive oil
Filling:
6 celery sticks, coarsely
  chopped
100 g (4 oz) button
  mushrooms, chopped
50 g (2 oz) unsalted, skinned
  peanuts, roughly chopped
½ teaspoon dried oregano
freshly ground black pepper
2 tablespoons chopped fresh
  parsley

PREPARATION TIME:
25 minutes, plus standing
COOKING TIME:
about 25 minutes
CALORIES PER PORTION:
255 (1065 kilojoules)

1. Mix the flour and salt in
a bowl; make a well in the
centre, and add the egg
and the milk plus water.
Beat until smooth and stir
in the parsley. Cover and
leave for 20 minutes.
2. Heat 1 tablespoon of oil
in a frying pan and fry the
celery for 3–4 minutes.
3. Add the mushrooms,
peanuts, oregano and
pepper and cook for 4–5
minutes. Stir in parsley.
4. Brush the base of a small
frying pan with oil. When
hot add sufficient batter to
thinly cover the base; cook
until golden on both sides.
Cook 7 more pancakes.
5. Divide the filling
between the pancakes, roll
them up, and serve.

FROM THE TOP Chilli beef; Smoked
haddock and celery risotto; Pancakes
with celery and peanuts

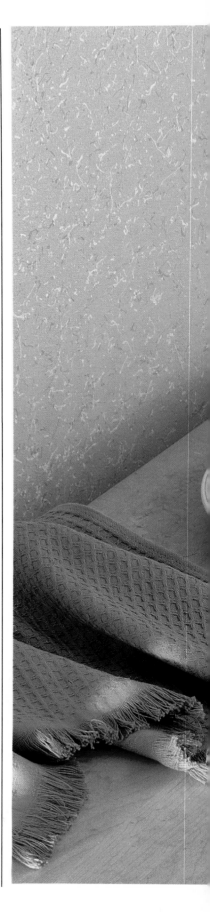

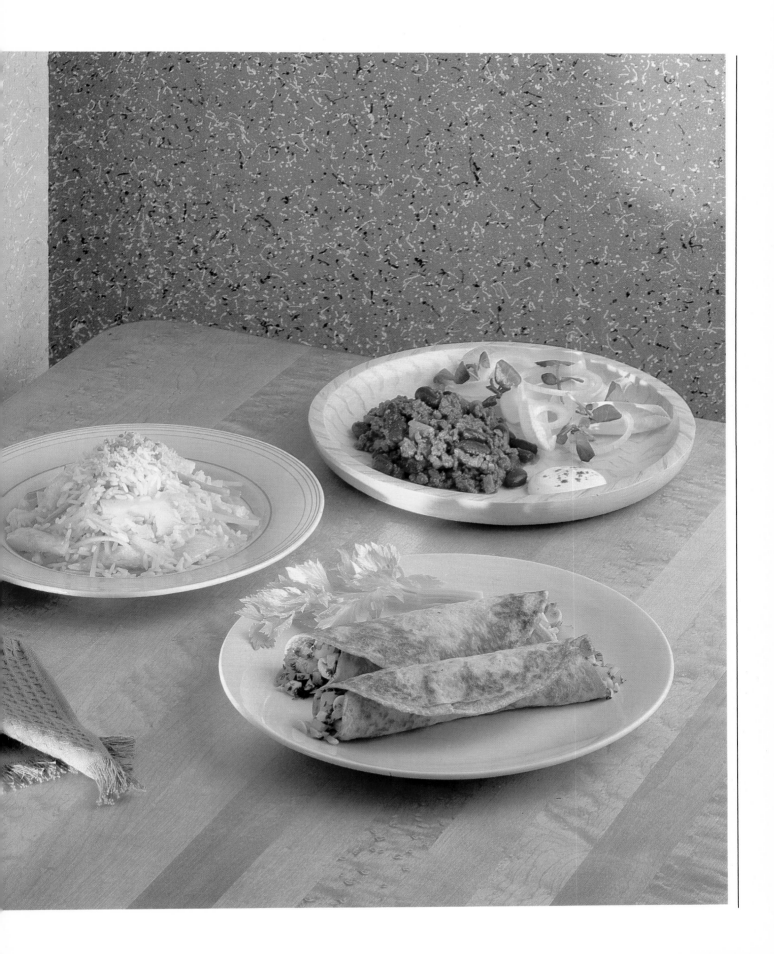

FEBRUARY

Puddings

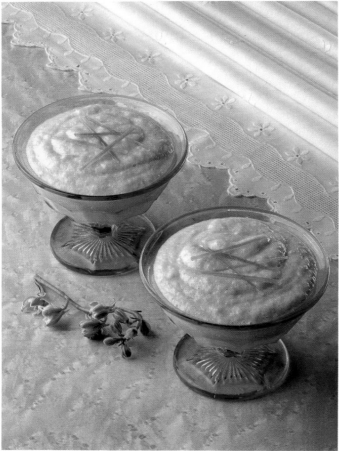

Snow Apple

450 g (1 lb) cooking apples,
  peeled, cored and sliced
3 tablespoons cider
2 tablespoons lemon curd
1 tablespoon ground almonds
2 eggs, separated
very fine strips of angelica, to
  decorate

PREPARATION TIME:
*20–25 minutes, plus cooling and
chilling*
COOKING TIME:
6 minutes
CALORIES PER PORTION:
140 (585 kilojoules)

1. Put the sliced apples and cider into a heavy based pan; cover the pan and simmer until the apple is soft and pulpy.
2. Beat the cooked apple to a purée and stir in the lemon curd, ground almonds and egg yolks; leave to cool.
3. Whisk the egg whites until stiff but not dry; fold lightly but thoroughly into the apple mixture.
4. Spoon into stemmed glasses and chill for 1 hour before serving, decorated with strips of angelica.

Stuffed Fresh Apricots

8 large ripe apricots
6 tablespoons orange juice
4 tablespoons dry white wine
225 g (8 oz) cottage cheese,
  sieved
1 banana, peeled and mashed
2 tablespoons lemon juice
pinch of ground cinnamon
2 teaspoons honey
fresh bay leaves (if available),
  to decorate (optional)

PREPARATION TIME:
about 35 minutes
CALORIES PER PORTION:
100 (420 kilojoules)

If you prefer to leave the apricots unskinned, start the method at step 2.

1. Nick the skin at the stalk end of each apricot; put into a bowl and cover with boiling water. Leave for 45 seconds then remove the apricots with a slotted spoon and carefully slip off the skins.
2. Halve the apricots, removing the stones, and put into a shallow dish; spoon over the orange juice and white wine.
3. Mix the sieved cottage cheese with the mashed banana, lemon juice, cinnamon and honey.
4. Lift out the apricot halves and arrange on a serving plate (or plates); fill each apricot half with the cheese mixture.
5. Spoon over a little of the orange and wine juices and decorate with fresh bay leaves if liked.

Lychee and Tangerine Salad

6 tangerines, peeled
150 ml (¼ pint) dry white
  wine
12 lychees, peeled
citrus leaves, sprigs of fresh
  mint or tiny fresh bay leaves,
  to decorate

PREPARATION TIME:
about 30 minutes
CALORIES PER PORTION:
230 (960 kilojoules)

1. Carefully remove the pith from each segment of tangerine; discard any pips.
2. Put one-third of the tangerine segments into a liquidizer with the white wine; blend until smooth.
3. Put 3 lychees into the centre of each small plate; arrange the remaining tangerine segments decoratively around the lychees.
4. Spoon the tangerine sauce over and around the fruits.
5. Decorate with citrus leaves, sprigs of mint or fresh bay leaves and serve.

LEFT Snow apple RIGHT, FROM TOP Stuffed fresh apricots; Lychee and tangerine salad

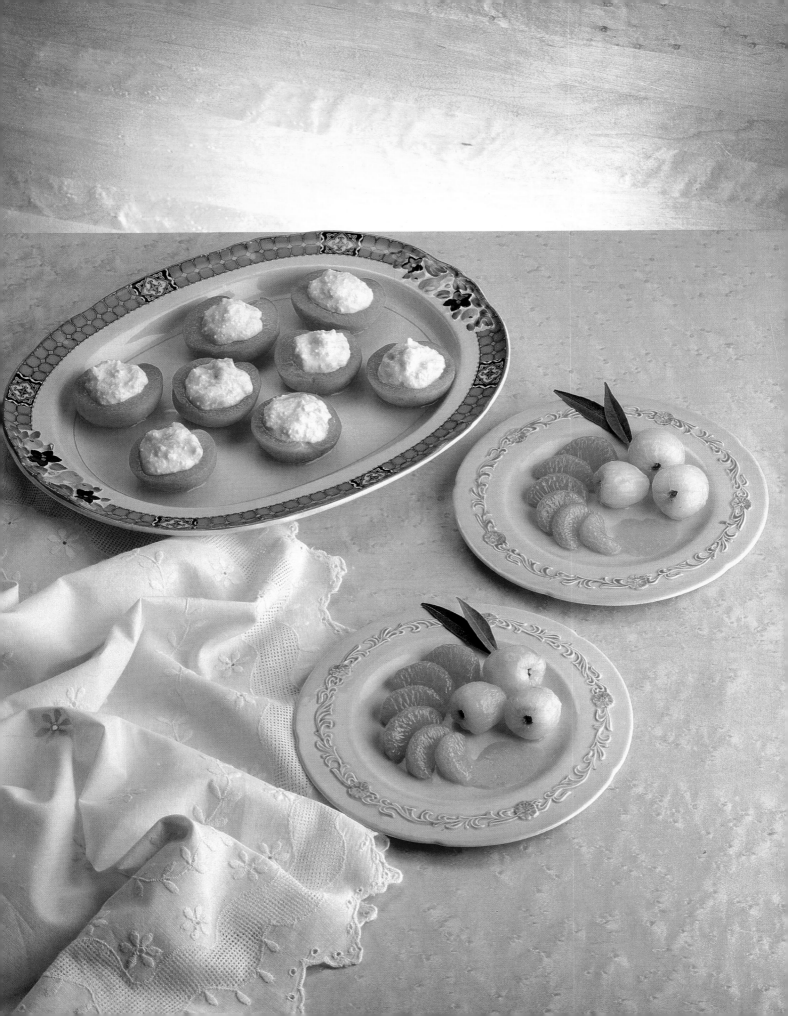

FEBRUARY

Dinner Party for Six

Mackerel and Mushrooms in Straw and Hay

350 g (12 oz) fresh paglia e fieno *pasta (see below)*
1 teaspoon olive oil
1 smoked mackerel fillet, flaked
225 g (8 oz) button mushrooms, sliced
salt
1 tablespoon lemon juice
1 garlic clove, peeled and very finely chopped
freshly ground black pepper

PREPARATION TIME:
15 minutes
COOKING TIME:
3–5 minutes
CALORIES PER PORTION:
155 (650 kilojoules)

Straw and hay is the translation of *paglia e fieno*, a very fine green and white pasta usually sold fresh, and the cooking time is for fresh pasta.

1. Cook the pasta in plenty of fast boiling salted water for 3–5 minutes until *al dente*.
2. Drain the pasta and immediately mix in the oil. Stir in all the other ingredients; cover and let the flavours mingle in the warmth of the pasta. Allow to cool.
3. Just before serving, taste and adjust the seasoning.

Poussin with Peas

18 very small onions, shallots, or large spring onions
1 tablespoon olive oil
3 garlic cloves, peeled and very finely chopped
3 fresh poussins, halved down the backbone
175 ml (6 fl oz) dry white wine
350 ml (12 fl oz) hot water
salt
freshly ground black pepper
1 kg (2 lb) peas

PREPARATION TIME:
20 minutes
COOKING TIME:
about 45 minutes
CALORIES PER PORTION:
270 (1130 kilojoules)

1. Peel the onions.
2. Heat the oil in a large heavy-based pan and fry the garlic and onions. When they have turned light golden remove.
3. Fry the poussins, turning frequently until sealed and browned all over, then add the wine. As soon as it boils, add the water and salt and pepper to taste.
4. Cover and simmer for 20 minutes, then uncover and simmer for another 20 minutes, adding the peas and onions about 8 minutes before cooking is completed.

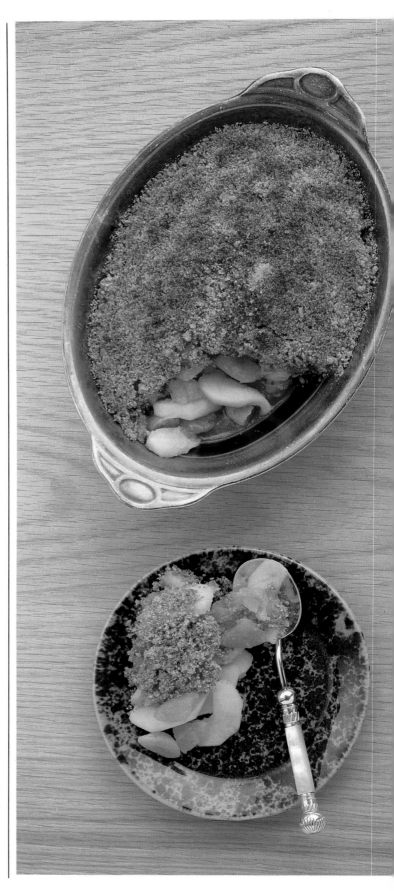

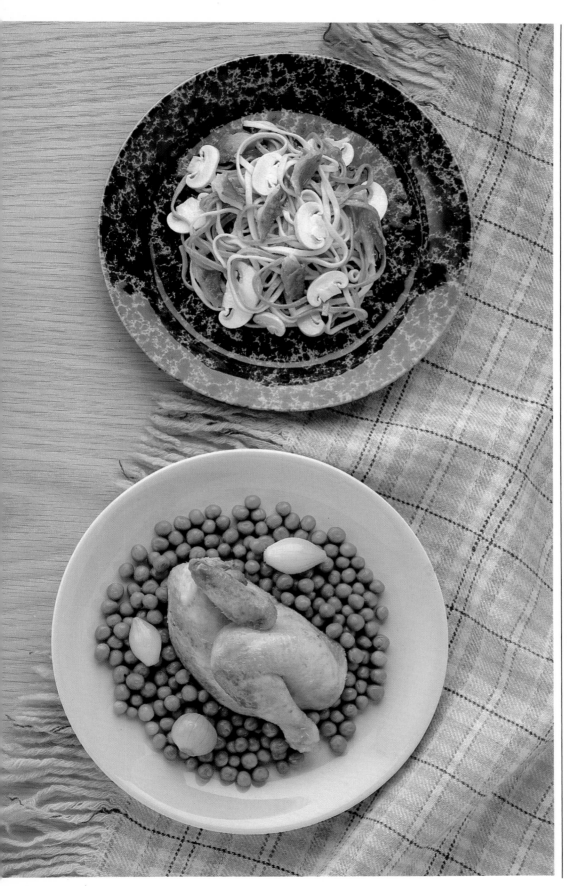

Apple and Apricot Wholemeal Crumble

750 g (1½ lb) tart eating apples, peeled, cored and chopped
1 tablespoon lemon juice
1 tablespoon water
175 g (6 oz) dried apricots, soaked overnight and chopped
½ teaspoon ground nutmeg
50 g (2 oz) butter
100 g (4 oz) wholemeal flour
25 g (1 oz) molasses sugar

PREPARATION TIME:
20 minutes, plus soaking
COOKING TIME:
1 hour
OVEN TEMPERATURE:
180°C, 350°F, Gas Mark 4
CALORIES PER PORTION:
225 (950 kilojoules)

1. Mix the apples with the lemon juice, water, apricots and nutmeg. Transfer to an ovenproof dish and press down well.
2. Work the butter into the flour with your fingers, then add the sugar a little at a time. When the texture resembles breadcrumbs, spread it lightly over the fruit.
3. Place in a preheated oven for about 1 hour. Allow to cool slightly before serving.

CLOCKWISE FROM TOP LEFT Apple and apricot wholemeal crumble; Mackerel and mushrooms in straw and hay; Poussin with peas

Side Salads

Celeriac with Lemon-Mustard Dressing

½ teaspoon mustard powder
3 tablespoons lemon juice
½ teaspoon clear honey
¼ teaspoon freshly ground
 black pepper
150 ml (¼ pint) plain
 unsweetened yogurt
pinch of salt
450 g (1 lb) peeled celeriac
1 carrot, coarsely shredded
¼ teaspoon paprika

PREPARATION TIME:
10 minutes
CALORIES PER SERVING:
about 85 (355 kilojoules)

The unattractive knobbly exterior of celeriac hides a distinctive and delicious celery-like flavour, which blends perfectly with lemon and mustard.

1. Blend together the mustard, lemon juice, honey, pepper, yogurt and salt and pour into a shallow serving dish.
2. Shred the celeriac very coarsely directly into the mixture to prevent discoloration. Stir in the carrot.
3. Sprinkle with the paprika and serve.

Red and White Salad

225 g (8 oz) fresh beetroot,
 scrubbed
225 g (8 oz) eating apple,
 washed
about 2 tablespoons lemon
 juice
2 chicory heads, cut into 1 cm
 (½ inch) thick slices
150 ml (¼ pint) plain
 unsweetened yogurt or
 cultured buttermilk
¼ teaspoon pepper
½–1 teaspoon mild mustard
pinch of salt
2 teaspoons sunflower oil

PREPARATION TIME:
5 minutes
COOKING TIME:
about 50 minutes
CALORIES PER SERVING:
about 85 (360 kilojoules)

If chicory is unavailable, use diced Chinese leaves instead.

1. Boil or steam the beetroot for about 50 minutes until tender. Drain and dice.
2. Quarter and core the apple then cut into small cubes. Toss in the lemon juice immediately to avoid discoloration.
3. Mix the apple with the chicory in a serving dish.
4. Combine the yogurt or buttermilk, pepper, mustard, salt and oil in a jug. Spoon over the salad.
5. Stir in the beetroot just before serving, as its colour will quickly stain the other salad ingredients.

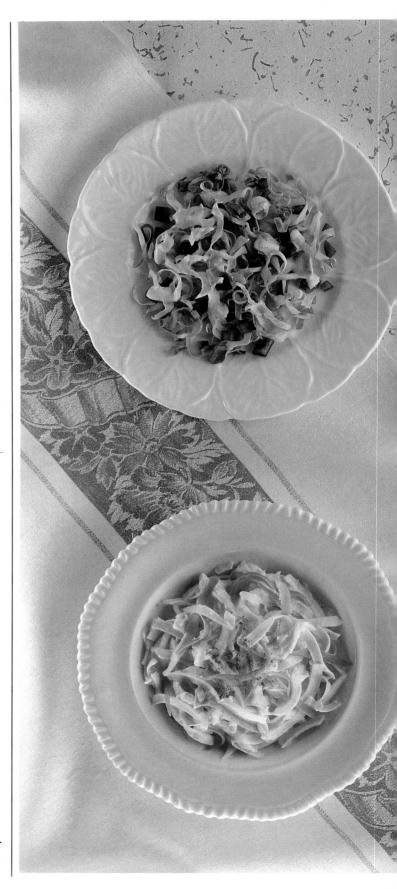

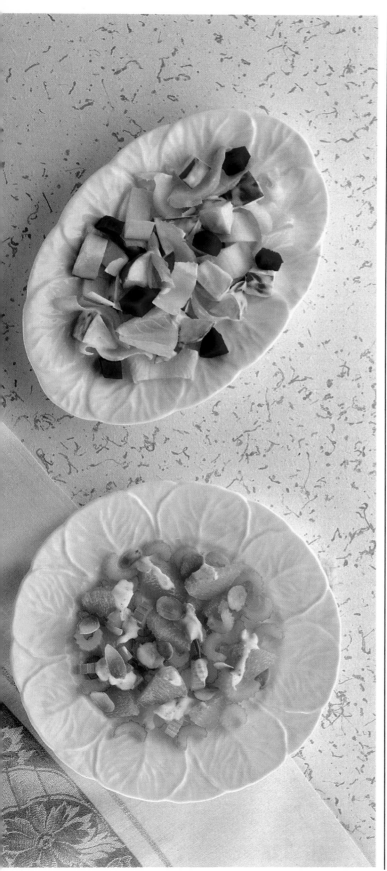

Crisp Winter Salad

40 g (1½ oz) flaked almonds
225 g (8 oz) celery, thinly
  sliced
1 large orange, about 175 g
  (6 oz) flesh, peeled,
  segmented and roughly
  chopped
150 ml (¼ pint) plain
  unsweetened yogurt
1 teaspoon ground coriander
  (optional)
½ teaspoon ground cumin or
  fennel seed
pinch of salt (optional)

PREPARATION TIME:
8 minutes
CALORIES PER SERVING:
about 100 (420 kilojoules)

A crunchy combination of
textures, sweetened with
orange and spices, makes
this salad a contrast to the
stodgy nature of much
winter food.

1. Place the almonds in an
ungreased heavy-based
frying pan over a low heat
for 2–3 minutes, stirring
until slightly browned.
2. Put half the almonds
with the prepared celery
and orange in a serving
bowl and toss lightly.
3. Combine the yogurt,
coriander (if using) and
cumin or fennel seed. Pour
over the salad. Taste and
add a little salt if necessary.
4. Sprinkle the remaining
almonds over the salad and
serve.

Savoy Salad

1 teaspoon caraway seeds
2 tablespoons olive or
  sunflower oil
2 teaspoons lemon juice
1 teaspoon red wine vinegar
1 teaspoon mild mustard
pinch of pepper
pinch of salt
100 g (4 oz) cottage or smooth
  low fat soft cheese
2 tablespoons water
225 g (8 oz) Savoy cabbage,
  very finely shredded
100 g (4 oz) red or green
  pepper, cored, seeded and
  finely diced

PREPARATION TIME:
10 minutes, plus standing
CALORIES PER SERVING:
about 115 (480 kilojoules)

The crinkly texture of
Savoy cabbage gives a fresh
look to this winter salad.
Cabbage and caraway are
traditional and
complementary partners.

1. Place the caraway seeds
in an ungreased heavy-
based frying pan and stir
over a low heat for 1–2
minutes. Crush in an
electric coffee mill or with
a mortar and pestle.
2. Transfer to a liquidizer
and add the oil, lemon
juice, vinegar, mustard,
pepper, salt, cheese and
water. Blend until smooth.
3. Place the prepared
cabbage and pepper in a
serving bowl and stir well.
4. Spoon the dressing over
and serve.

CLOCKWISE FROM TOP LEFT Savoy
salad: Red and white salad; Crisp
winter salad; Celeriac with lemon-
mustard dressing

WINTER

Main Course Salads

Cottage Coleslaw

*225 g (8 oz) white cabbage,
  finely shredded*
*225 g (8 oz) carrots, coarsely
  shredded*
3 sticks celery, finely sliced
*1 bunch watercress, base of
  stems removed, chopped*
*100 g (4 oz) green-skinned
  apple, diced*
*2 teaspoons lemon or orange
  juice*
50 g (2 oz) sultanas
*50 g (2 oz) hazelnuts, toasted
  and chopped*
*150 ml (¼ pint) plain
  unsweetened yogurt*
1 teaspoon wine vinegar
*½ teaspoon dried tarragon or
  crushed caraway seeds*
pinch of salt
large pinch of pepper
450 g (1 lb) cottage cheese

PREPARATION TIME:
15 minutes
CALORIES PER SERVING:
about 260 (2200 kilojoules)

The calorie count here is
low enough for you to add
1–2 tablespoons low
calorie dressing if you like.

1. Mix all the ingredients
except the cottage cheese
in a large bowl, making
sure the apple is quickly
coated in the lemon or
orange juice.
2. Spoon the cottage
cheese on to the other
ingredients in the bowl
and mix well. Serve
immediately.

Seafood Salad

*225 g (8 oz) potatoes, washed
  but not peeled*
350 g (12 oz) white fish
150 ml (¼ pint) boiling water
100 g (4 oz) shelled prawns
*½ bunch watercress, base of
  stems removed, chopped*
*½ head endive or crisp
  lettuce, torn into small pieces*
1 carrot, coarsely shredded
*2 tablespoons chopped fresh
  parsley*
*150 ml (¼ pint) plain
  unsweetened yogurt*
2 teaspoons walnut or olive oil
pinch of salt
*1–2 tablespoons chopped fresh
  dill*
*2 hard-boiled eggs, cut into
  wedges*

PREPARATION TIME:
10 minutes
COOKING TIME:
25 minutes
CALORIES PER SERVING:
about 250 (1045 kilojoules)

The model for many
different variations, this
salad can be made with
any type of white fish
(even smoked cod) and
using sliced scallops,
mussels, crabmeat or
winkles instead of prawns.
Cooked leeks make a good
alternative to potatoes.

1. Boil or steam the
potatoes until just tender,
about 20 minutes. Drain
and dice.
2. Poach the fish gently in
the boiling water for 5
minutes in a covered pan.
Cool then break into bite-
size pieces.
3. Combine the potatoes,
fish, prawns, watercress,
endive or lettuce, carrot
and parsley in a serving
dish.
4. Liquidize the yogurt
with the oil, salt and dill.
Stir into the salad, and
taste to check the
seasoning.
5. Serve, accompanied by
the wedges of hard-boiled
egg.

Curried Butterbean Salad

*350 g (12 oz) butterbeans,
  soaked overnight*
2 teaspoons vegetable oil
*2 onions, peeled and finely
  chopped*
2 teaspoons curry powder
*150 ml (¼ pint) plain
  unsweetened yogurt*
1 tablespoon lemon juice
pinch of salt
pinch of pepper
To serve:
½ lettuce, washed (optional)
*1 sprig fresh rosemary to
  garnish, if available*

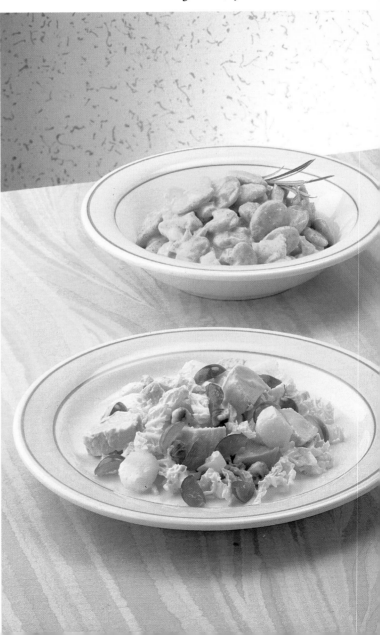

PREPARATION TIME:
12 minutes plus soaking
COOKING TIME:
1 hour 10 minutes
CALORIES PER SERVING:
about 305 (1280 kilojoules)

Butterbeans, like other pulses, provide plenty of protein for a main course – and they're very filling too.

1. Drain the butterbeans from their soaking water, put in a large pan, cover with fresh water and bring to the boil. Cover and simmer for 1 hour, or until tender but not broken. Drain.

2. Heat the oil in a heavy-based pan, add the onions and cook gently for 8 minutes, covering the pan. Add the curry powder and cook for a further 2 minutes.
3. Meanwhile, mix the yogurt with the lemon juice, salt and pepper.
4. Add this to the onion mixture, then stir in the butterbeans.
5. To serve, arrange a bed of lettuce on a serving plate, if using, spoon the butterbeans on top and garnish with a sprig of rosemary.

Turkey Salad

50 g (2 oz) hazelnuts
75 g (3 oz) grapes, quartered and pipped
100 g (4 oz) drained canned water chestnuts
225 g (8 oz) Chinese leaves, finely shredded
450 g (1 lb) cooked turkey meat, cut in bite-size pieces

Dressing:
3 teaspoons grated Parmesan cheese
1 egg
2 teaspoons olive, sunflower or walnut oil
2 teaspoons lemon or orange juice
pinch of English mustard powder
1 clove garlic, peeled and crushed (optional)
pinch of freshly ground black pepper
pinch of sea salt
few drops of Worcestershire sauce
150 ml (¼ pint) plain unsweetened yogurt

PREPARATION TIME:
15 minutes
CALORIES PER SERVING:
about 325 (1360 kilojoules)

Turkey is a very lean meat, so keep cooked turkey from becoming too dry by refrigerating it in stock.

1. Place the hazelnuts in an ungreased heavy-based pan over a low heat for 2–3 minutes, stirring until lightly browned.
2. Combine with all the other salad ingredients in a large bowl.
3. Blend all the dressing ingredients except the yogurt in a liquidizer. Transfer to a jug.
4. Mix the yogurt into the dressing by hand and stir the dressing into the salad. Mix well then serve.

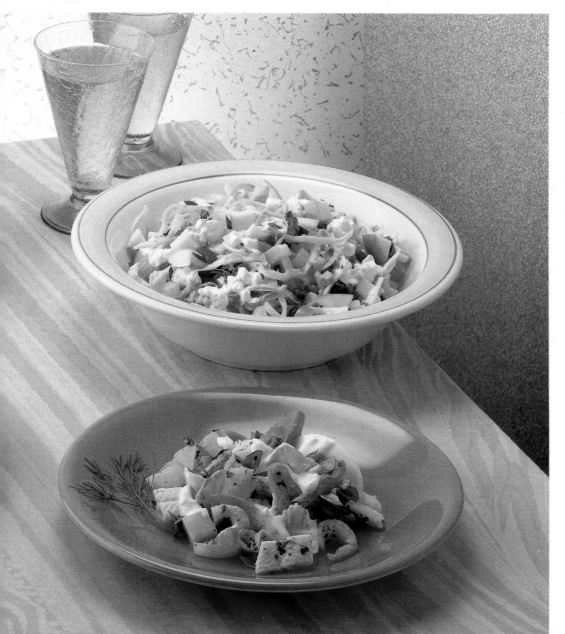

CLOCKWISE FROM TOP LEFT
Curried butterbean salad; Cottage coleslaw; Seafood salad; Turkey salad

INDEX

Photography: Vernon Morgan **Photographic styling:** Penny Mishcon and Carolyn Russell
Preparation of food for photography: Allyson Birch and Anne Ager
Cover illustration: Patricia MacCarthy
The publishers would like to thank the following companies for the loan of props for photography:
David Mellor, 4 Sloane Square, London SW1; Elizabeth David, 46 Bourne Street,
London SW1
Designers Guild, 277 King's Road, London SW3; Souleiado, 171 Fulham Road,
London SW3
H.K. Williamson Veneers, Unit 29, Staffa Industrial Estate, Staffa Road, Leyton,
London E10